Binocular Vision Anomalies

INVESTIGATION AND TREATMENT

Second edition

David Pickwell, MSc, FBOA HD, FBCO, D,Orth
Professor of Optometry, Department of Optometry, University of Bradford

BUTTERWORTH
HEINEMANN

Butterworth–Heinemann Ltd
Halley Court, Jordan Hill, Oxford OX2 8EJ

PART OF REED INTERNATIONAL P.L.C.

OXFORD LONDON GUILDFORD BOSTON MUNICH NEWDELHI
SINGAPORE SYDNEY TOKYO TORONTO WELLINGTON

First published 1984
Second edition, 1989
Reprinted 1991

British Library Cataloguing in Publication Data

Pickwell, David
Binocular vision anomalies.—2nd ed.
1. Man. Binocular vision disorders
I. Title
617.7′62

ISBN 0 7506 1488 9

Library of Congress Cataloging-in-Publication Data

Pickwell, David.
Binocular vision anomalies: investigation and treatment/ David Pickwell.—2nd ed.
p. cm.
Includes bibliographies and index.
ISBN 0 7506 1488 9
1. Binocular vision disorders. I. Title
[DNLM: 1. Eye Diseases—diagnosis. 2. Eye Diseases—therapy. 3.Orthoptics. WW 405 P597b]
RE735.P53 1989
617.7′62—dc19

Composition by Genesis Typesetting, Laser Quay, Rochester, Kent
Printed and bound by Hartnolls Ltd, Bodmin, Cornwall

Preface

This second edition is intended as an update of the original book on the practical and clinical aspects of binocular vision for students and practitioners. The 'how-to-do-it' approach has been retained and in some cases extended. The theory of binocular vision has been kept to the minimum necessary to understand the investigative and therapeutic procedures.

The approach to heterophoria has been developed in this edition and the emphasis on evaluating the level of compensation and stability rather than phoria measurements has been amplified in the light of more recent clinical research in this area.

A new summary chapter on the evaluation and management of squint has been added. This describes a practical classification of squint in terms of which types can be treated by non-surgical methods and it indicates the methods found to be successful in the experience of the author. This has made redundant a previous chapter on prescribing and prognosis, but the details of the methods of treatment are contained in the earlier chapters as in the previous edition.

New material has been added to the chapter on pre-school-age children to help the understanding of departures from normal visual development. This is linked with an indication of which investigative methods are appropriate at each age in deciding if normal development has occurred.

Again I wish to acknowledge the contributions of my colleagues who share in the binocular vision clinic at Bradford University, and those who have recently collaborated in the research work. In particular I acknowledge Dr T.C.A. Jenkins, Mr J.M. Gilchrist and Dr A.A. Yekta. I also express my thanks to the staff of Butterworths for their real interest in the progress of this book.

D.P.

Preface to First Edition

This book is intended to provide a clinical text on the investigation and management of binocular vision anomalies by methods other than medicine and surgery. It is hoped that it will be useful to the student facing the subject for the first time, and also to the established practitioner seeking a reference to the binocular anomalies likely to be seen in everyday practice. The aim has been to produce a 'how-to-do-it' book. It is not a textbook on the theory of binocular vision. There are a number of excellent books which cover the anatomy, physiology and mechanisms of binocular vision. The theory has therefore been kept to the minimum necessary for an adequate appreciation of the anomalies, their investigation and treatment. I have assumed that the reader has a basic knowledge of normal binocular vision or is acquiring this simultaneously with clinical studies. I also assume a knowledge of the general procedures of eye examination and refractive methods.

The history and past literature of orthoptics seems to be full of descriptions of unsubstantiated methods which have come and gone as it was found that they did not work. At times it has appeared to have been a maze of suggested procedures which have varied from 'cure-alls' to useful clinical ideas. I cannot claim to have explored all of them. What I have tried to do is describe the methods which I have found effective, and where possible provided the references for practical evaluations. I have tried to write from my own particular experience which has extended over thirty years. In doing so, I am very aware of others whose experience has been parallel, but not necessarily the same. As far as possible, I have also tried to reflect some of their views, and acknowledge their contributions to the ongoing development of clinical practice.

To help the student, I have tried to provide a recognizable pattern in dealing with the conditions described, and I hope thereby to have produced a mnemonic approach to the subject which will aid learning and application in a clinical setting. Each condition is dealt with in the general order of definition, investigation, evaluation and management. Under the heading of management, I have considered five non-medical possibilities: removing any general cause, correcting refractive error, orthoptics, relieving prisms and referral. These patterns will be obvious in the early chapters, and are assumed in the later ones.

I wish particularly to acknowledge the work and encouragement given to me by my colleagues in the binocular vision clinics at the University of Bradford, who have stimulated my thoughts and actions over many years. I would mention Mr M. Sheridan and Dr W. A. Douthwaite. I am particularly indebted in this respect to Dr T. C. A. Jenkins who also read the manuscript and made many helpful suggestions. I wish to thank Mrs J. Paley for interpreting the initial draft and for typing the manuscript, and also the staff of the Graphics Unit of the University of Bradford for their help with the illustrations.

D.P.

Contents

Part I

Investigation

1

Nature of binocular vision anomalies

Introduction

Binocular vision is the co-ordination and integration of what is received from the two eyes separately into a single binocular percept. Proper functioning of binocular vision without symptoms depends on a number of factors which can be considered under three broad headings:

(1) The anatomy of the visual apparatus.
(2) The motor system that co-ordinates movement of the eyes.
(3) The sensory system whereby the brain receives and integrates the two monocular perceptions.

Anomalies in any of these can cause difficulties in binocular vision, or even make it impossible. In considering the binocular difficulties of a particular patient, therefore, all three parts of the total system need to be investigated:

(1) *Anatomy.* Abnormalities in the anatomy of the visual system can be either developmental or acquired. They can occur in the embryological development before birth of the bony orbit, ocular muscles or parts of the nervous system. Accident or disease can also change the anatomy.
(2) *Motor system.* Even if the motor system is anatomically normal, anomalies can occur in the functioning which can disturb binocular vision or cause it to break down. These may also be due to disease, or they may be malfunctions of the physiology of the motor system. For example, excessive accommodation due to uncorrected hyperopia can result in excessive convergence due to the accommodation–convergence relationship. This is a fairly frequent cause of binocular vision problems. When it occurs in young children, and if left untreated, it can result in a permanent breakdown in binocular vision. In adults, it can create disturbing symptoms. Examples of disease affecting the motor system are haemorrhages involving the nerve supply to the extrinsic muscles, local changes in intracranial pressure near the nerve nuclei or pressure on the nerves or nerve centres from abnormal growths of intracranial tissue. Such conditions require medical attention to the primary condition, rather than immediate treatment of the binocular anomaly. Early recognition of these

conditions is essential, and the investigation for this type of pathology is dealt with more fully in Chapter 16.

(3) *Sensory system.* Anomalies in the sensory system can arise from such factors as a loss of clarity of the optical image in one or both eyes, an image larger in one eye than the other (aniseikonia), anomalies of the visual pathway or cortex, or central factors in the integrating mechanism. Difficulties in the co-ordinating mechanism of the motor system can also be accompanied by adaptations in the sensory system, such as suppression, abnormal correspondence or amblyopia. These occur in order to lessen the symptoms caused by the motor anomaly, but are adaptations of the sensory system.

The anatomical, motor and sensory aspects need to be normal if normal binocular vision is to be present. The position of the eyes relative to each other is determined first by their anatomical position. Humans have forward-looking eyes placed in the front of the skull, and this brings the visual axes of the two eyes almost parallel to each other. In most cases, they are slightly divergent when the position is determined only by anatomical factors, and this is known as the *position of anatomical rest*. In normal circumstances, this state seldom exists, as physiological factors are nearly always operative also. These factors, such as the tonus of the muscles and the sensed direction or distance of the objects under view, usually make the visual axes less divergent – the *position of physiological rest*. Included in the physiological factors affecting the position of the eyes is the accommodation–convergence relationship: the eyes will converge as accommodation is exerted, and this is usually known as *accommodative convergence*. The final adjustment of the eyes is made in the interests of single binocular vision. This is traditionally known as *fusional convergence*, and brings the retinal images on corresponding points (or within Panum's areas). For distance vision, this will produce parallel visual axes.

If the fusional aspect is suspended, for example, by covering one eye, the position of the eyes will be determined only by the anatomical and physiological factors. Usually this *dissociated position* is slightly deviated from the *active position* which is maintained when all of the factors are free to operate. This slight deviation from the active position when the eyes are dissociated is known as *heterophoria*; sometimes abbreviated to phoria. It is present in most people. Very rarely, it is not present, that is, the dissociated position is the same as the active position, and this is known as *orthophoria*. It needs to be appreciated that the term 'heterophoria' applies only to the deviation of the eyes that occurs when the fusional factor is prevented by covering one eye or dissociated by other methods such as distorting one eye's image so that it cannot be fused with the other, e.g. the Maddox rod method (see Chapter 3). Heterophoria is often considered to be a latent deviation; it only becomes manifest on dissociation of the two eyes. Sometimes the eyes can be deviated even when no dissociation is introduced. This more permanent deviation is called *heterotropia, squint* or *strabismus*. Ocular deviations, then, can be classified as either heterophoria or squint, but there are other important practical classifications that need to be considered in investigating the binocular vision of a patient.

Most binocular vision anomalies fit into a recognized pattern, which is to say that experience has taught that patients can be grouped according to a similarity of the symptoms and clinical features. Discovering the pattern into which a particular patient fits is the process of *diagnosis* and is the obvious preliminary to treatment. The classifications adopted here are intended to assist diagnosis (see *Figure 1.1*).

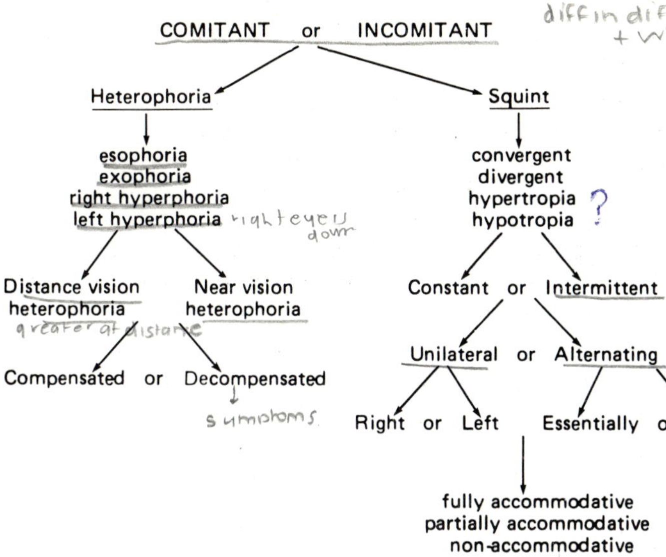

Figure 1.1. Classification of ocular deviations

Comitancy

Ocular deviations can be classified as comitant or incomitant. Comitant deviations are the same in all directions of gaze for a particular distance of fixation. Incomitant deviations vary with the direction of gaze; that is, as the patient moves the eyes to fix objects in different parts of the motor field, the degree or the angle of the deviation will vary. For example, the deviation may be more when the patient is looking up and to the left than in other parts of the field. There may be no deviation in one part of the motor field, but a marked deviation in other parts. Incomitant deviations are also referred to as paralytic or paretic: a paresis is a partial paralysis. Usually they are caused by abnormalities of the anatomy or of the functioning of the motor system due to accident or disease, or of development. It is important to distinguish incomitant deviations from those that are comitant, as the treatment can be quite different and have different priorities. An incomitant deviation of sudden onset is usually caused by accident or active pathology requiring immediate medical attention.

Classification of heterophoria

Heterophoria can be classified in the clinical investigation by the direction of the deviation, by the fixation distance at which the heterophoria occurs, or whether it is compensated or not.

Direction of deviation

When the eyes are dissociated, the deviation that occurs can be in any direction, or may be a combination of more than one direction. Classification according to the direction of the deviation is as follows:

(1) *Esophoria* – visual axes convergent when the eyes are dissociated.
(2) *Exophoria* – visual axes divergent when the eyes are dissociated.
(3) *Hyperphoria* – visual axes vertically misaligned when the eyes are dissociated: if the right eye is higher than the left, it is 'right hyperphoria', and if the left eye is higher, 'left hyperphoria'.
(4) *Cyclophoria* – the eyes rotate about the visual axes when dissociated: if the top of the primary vertical meridian rotates nasally, it is called 'incyclophoria', and if it rotates temporally, 'excyclophoria'. It is doubtful whether cyclophoria exists as an isolated condition.

It should be noted that right hyperphoria is the same as a dissociated deviation of the left eye downwards. It can therefore be referred to as 'left hypophoria'. Similarly, left hyperphoria is the equivalent of 'right hypophoria'. In practice, the term 'hypophoria' is seldom used, these deviations being referred to as right or left hyperphoria.

Fixation distance

The second method of classifying heterophoria is according to the distance of fixation. This is usually either at 6 m, which is the distance used for testing the patient's distance vision, or at the distance the patient uses for near vision, which is usually 33–40 cm. These are known as the 'distance phoria' and 'near phoria', respectively, and they may differ in degree and direction from each other. The phoria may also have more clinical significance for one distance and not for the other; that is, it may cause symptoms only for distance vision or only for near visual tasks. It is therefore important to investigate the phoria at the distance for which the patient normally uses the eyes, and to discover if the symptoms are associated with vision at that distance.

With children and young adults, the degree of heterophoria is very much the same for distance and near vision, but from the mid-twenties, the average person slowly becomes more exophoric for near vision. The average phoria for distance vision remains the same, but at 65 years the near phoria has increased by 6^{Δ} (Δ = prism dioptres) (Freier and Pickwell, 1983). This exophoric difference for near vision is called 'physiological exophoria'.

Duane (1896) suggested a method of classification for squint based on whether the vergence was greater for distance or near vision. This is now applied in a modified form to heterophoria as well as squint. It is useful in relating the patient's symptoms to the actual problem, and also in selecting the most appropriate treatment.

(1) *Esophoria*
   (a) Divergence weakness esophoria – usually considered an anomaly of distance vision: the degree of esophoria is greater for distance than for near vision.
   (b) Convergence excess esophoria – a higher degree of esophoria for near vision than for distance.
   (c) Basic (or mixed) esophoria – the degree does not differ significantly with the fixation distance.
(2) *Exophoria*
   (a) Convergence weakness exophoria – a higher degree of exophoria for near vision than for distance.

(b) Divergence excess exophoria – a higher degree of deviation for distance vision than for near. This type often breaks down into a squint for distance fixation, and therefore may be considered to be an intermittent squint.
(c) Basic (or mixed) exophoria – the degree does not differ significantly with the fixation distance.
(d) Convergence insufficiency – an inability to maintain sufficient convergence for comfortable near vision. This may be considered an anomaly of convergence rather than heterophoria. It is often, but not always accompanied by convergence weakness exophoria.

Compensation

The third and clinically very important classification of heterophoria is as either compensated or decompensated (Marton, 1954). As already stated, heterophoria is a normal condition in that it is present in the vast majority of people. It is considered a physiological condition, as in most cases it gives no trouble and no symptoms. In these circumstances it is described as 'compensated'. Sometimes, however, there are abnormal stresses on the binocular vision which results in symptoms and the heterophoria becomes 'decompensated'. This is more likely to happen if there are developmental abnormalities in the anatomical, motor or sensory systems. These may not in themselves make the phoria decompensated, and in very many cases do not (Lyle and Wybar, 1967). A change in the patient's general or visual conditions may add additional stress, and symptoms can occur. Obviously, identifying these changes is an important part of the investigation of decompensated heterophoria. The first consideration in treatment is to remove as many as possible of the decompensating factors

The following factors may contribute to heterophoria becoming decompensated, particularly if there is a marked change in them:

STRESS ON THE VISUAL SYSTEM

(1) *Excessive use of vision under adverse circumstances*
(a) Work held too close to the eyes for long periods. A comfortable working distance depends on the amplitude of accommodation, and therefore on the patient's age. As the amplitude starts to decrease during the teenage years, stress on accommodation and convergence can occur if a proper working distance is not adopted. The near distance can also present stress in early presbyopia (Pickwell, Jenkins and Yekta, 1987).
(b) A sudden increase in the amount of close work. This can occur with a change of occupation; for example, students nearing examination time, or leaving school to start a clerical job.
(c) Poor illumination or contrast (Pickwell, Yekta and Jenkins, 1987). Although visual working conditions are usually controlled in factories, offices, schools, shops, etc., it may be necessary to give these some thought. Visual conditions in the home can be very variable. Bad ventilation can also contribute to visual stress.
(d) Increased use of the pursuit reflexes: for example; playing or watching ball-games, or reading in the unsteady conditions on some public transport.
(e) Night driving conditions may produce long periods of looking into a dark field with very reduced fusion stimulus at a time when the patient is fatigued.

(2) *Accommodative anomalies*. Because of the relationship of accommodation and convergence, anomalies of accommodation can put stress on binocular vision. The additional accommodation required by an uncorrected hyperope to get clear vision or the high accommodative effort in incipient presbyopia are examples of this. Both of these conditions may show decompensated phoria until the appropriate refractive correction is given.
(3) *Refractive error*. Other refractive errors – astigmatism and anisometropia (and sometimes myopia) – can make fusion more difficult due to the image blur being unequal between the two eyes and contribute to decompensation of the phoria.
(4) *Imbalanced prism vergences* (sometimes known as binocular ductions or fusional reserves; see Chapter 3). Where there is stress on the binocular vision, the prism vergences are often found to be imbalanced. It is not known if this is a cause of the stress or the result of it, but the prism vergences of individuals are known to vary from time to time.

STRESS ON THE WELL-BEING OF THE PATIENT

(1) *Poor general health*. A deterioration in the patient's health can result in decompensation of the phoria (Pickwell and Hampshire, 1984). This is particularly true if other decompensating factors are also present.
(2) *Worry and anxiety*. It is helpful to know if there are major worries that may contribute to the binocular vision symptoms, even if the problems themselves are not visual. If the situation is temporary, as with a student's pre-examination stress for example, this may affect the type or the timing of treatment. The treatment may be temporary in anticipation of a further visual examination and assessment when the other problems have been relieved.
(3) *Old age*. This can be important for decompensation of near phoria. The general loss of muscle strength with extreme age will also affect the compensation of phoria. Elderly patients do not respond well to orthoptic treatment and prism relief is considered.
(4) *Emotional and temperamental problems*. Psychological difficulties and personality problems are difficult to assess during a vision examination, but they may also be a factor. While these may be recognized, they lie outside the scope of binocular vision treatment, although it may be necessary to take them into account. However, their presence can be a useful reminder that we are not dealing just with eyes, but with people.
(5) *Adverse effect of medicines*. The side effects of medicinal drugs can rarely affect binocular vision directly. Some reduce the amplitude of accommodation, and can therefore affect binocular vision indirectly.

Classification of strabismus

As well as deciding whether strabismus or squint is comitant or incomitant, it can be classified according to constancy, eye preference and the direction of deviation. In some patients the angle varies with the accommodative state. Squints may also be present for both distance vision and for near vision, or at only one fixation distance. The angle of deviation may also vary with the fixation distance, giving classifications of divergence weakness, convergence excess or basic types of convergent squints; and convergence weakness, divergent excess or basic types of divergent squints. These correspond with the classifications of heterophoria (see above).

Constancy

Squint can be classified as either (1) constant or (2) intermittent. It is described as constant if it is present all the time and under all circumstances, and intermittent if it is present at some times and not at others. Some squints are intermittent in the sense that some patients have co-ordinated binocular vision most of the time, but when the visual system or general well-being is under stress the squint occurs. In these cases, binocular vision does not show the signs of decompensated heterophoria, but breaks down into a squint. In some cases, an intermittent squint will develop into a constant squint if left untreated, but in others it seems to remain intermittent. A rare form of intermittent squint is referred to as 'cyclic squint': Costenbader and Mousel (1964) found it to be less than than 0.1% of all squints. The patient has a large convergent squint on alternate days only. The cyclic squint usually becomes constant after a few months.

In the case of intermittent squint, it is useful to try to assess the proportion of time when the squint is present. A patient who has binocular vision for most of the time may have a better prognosis.

Direction of deviation

The classification by the direction of the deviation is illustrated in *Figure 1.2.*

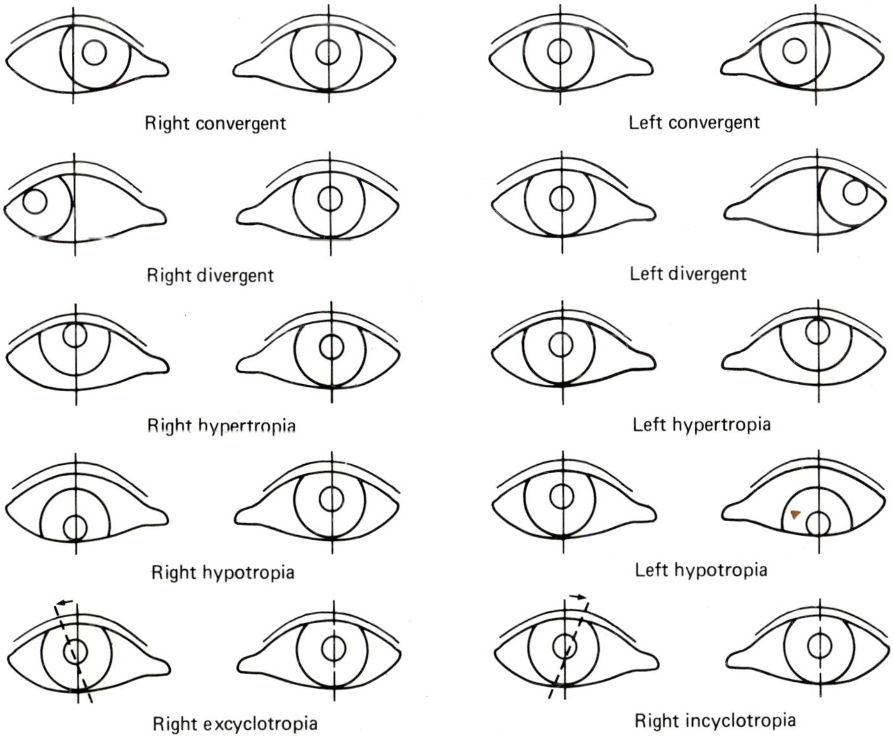

Figure 1.2. Classification of squint by direction of deviation

Eye preference

In squint, an image of the object of regard will be maintained on the fovea of one eye, while the other eye is deviated. Some patients always use the same eye for fixation, and others can fix with either eye. Squint then can be classified as (1) unilateral or (2) alternating. Obviously, a unilateral squint can be either a right eye or a left eye squint depending on which eye is deviated.

In alternating squint, the eye chosen for fixation at any given time can depend on:

(a) Fixation distance. Some patients will use one eye for distance vision and the other for near.
(b) Direction of gaze. In some patients the eye used for fixation will depend on the direction of gaze. In convergent squint, this often indicates a congenital impairment in the abducting function of one or both eyes. The right eye fixes objects in the left of the field, and the left eye in the right; this is known as 'crossed fixation'.
(c) Vision and refraction. If the vision and the refractive error are equal or nearly equal, the choice of eye for fixation may appear indiscriminate. Some cases of this type are considered to lack the ability to fuse, and these have been called 'essentially alternating' (Worth, 1903). These are often divergent squints, and do not respond to treatment to establish binocular vision. Some other alternating squints will become unilateral if left untreated.

Accommodative state

The angle of the squint may vary with the amount of accommodation exerted. In hyperopes this is an important factor in the treatment, so that squint may be classified as: (1) fully accommodative, (2) partially accommodative or (3) non-accommodative.

It is estimated that about two-thirds of comitant convergent squint has an accommodative element. This means that the angle will be reduced by a refractive correction for hyperopia; fully in some cases, and partially in others. In such cases, the spectacle correction forms a major part of the treatment of the deviation.

In about one-third of comitant convergent squint, the spectacle correction does not change the angle of deviation. These are the non-accommodative squints. However, it needs to be appreciated that some patients with non-accommodative squint will over-converge for near vision. In these cases, the convergence excess is not stimulated by the accommodative effort.

Importance of classification

In the clinical assessment of both heterophoria and squint, the classification will assist in deciding what can be done to help the patient; the clinical management.

In cases of heterophoria, for example, it will be appreciated that most important is whether the deviation is compensated or not; if there are symptoms present. Clearly symptom free heterophoria may require no action unless there are other anomalies present such as the suppression of one eye. The management of esophoria is different from that of exophoria. It will also differ if the heterophoria is present for near vision as accommodation is normally active compared to distance vision when little accommodation will be in play for fully corrected eyes.

In the same way, the management of squint will depend first on the classification. This is further elaborated in chapter 15.

References

COSTENBADER, F. D. and MOUSEL, D. K. (1964). Cyclic esotropia. *Archives of Ophthalmology*, **71**, 180–183

DUANE, A. (1896). A new classification of the motor anomalies of the eyes based upon physiological principles. *Annals of Ophthalmology*, **5**, 969; **6**, 251

FREIER, B. E. and PICKWELL, L. D. (1983). Physiological exophoria. *Ophthalmic and Physiological Optics*, **3**, 267–272

LYLE, T. K. and WYBAR, K. C. (1967). *Practical Orthoptics in the Tratment of Squint*. H. K. Lewis, London, p. 424

MARTON, H. B. (1954). Some clinical aspects of heterophoria. *British Journal of Physiological Optics*, **11**(3), 170–175

PICKWELL, L. D. and HAMPSHIRE, R. (1984). Convergence insufficiency in patients taking medicines. *Ophthalmic and Physiological Optics*, **4**, 151–154

PICKWELL, D., JENKINS, T. C. A. and YEKTA, A. A. (1987). The effect of fixation disparity and associated heterophoria of reading at an abnormally close distance. *Ophthalmic and Physiological Optics*, **7**(4), 345–347

PICKWELL, L. D., YEKTA, A. A. and JENKINS, T. C. A. (1987). The effect of reading in low illumination on fixation disparity. *American Journal of Optometry*, **64**(7), 513–518

WORTH, C. (1903). *Squint*. Baillière, Tindall & Cox, London

2

Binocular vision in routine examination

The routine for examining the eyes and vision of every patient should have two objectives: to detect the presence of all the anomalies that might be expected and/or to indicate when further investigative tests are required. In some cases the patient will indicate by the presenting symptoms or history that a binocular anomaly is likely to be the cause of the trouble. With other patients, binocular vision anomalies will be discovered during the examination, although these were not obvious to the patient. The routine examination should also indicate whether to proceed with further investigation, with treatment, or to refer for medical attention.

An outline of the routine procedures is illustrated in *Figure 2.1*. It will be seen that the type of investigation of the binocular functions will depend on whether a squint or heterophoria has been found. Whereas a routine examination will have broader objectives, the following description emphasizes particularly the binocular vision aspects.

Preliminary details

These will include such information as the name and address. More important, clinically, is the age of the patient. This must be noted in relation to the age of onset of any squint, as it is likely to affect the extent of the sensory adaptations and the prognosis.

The patient's occupation should also be noted, so that the visual conditions of work and recreational activities are understood. Some patients have a greater need for stereopsis, and others use their eyes in conditions that put a greater stress on binocular vision. Changes in occupation can also help in understanding the cause of the patient's problem.

History and symptoms

It is to be expected that many patients will attend for examination at regular intervals, although they are not complaining of symptoms. This can result in the early detection of any anomalies. Symptoms often occur at an advanced stage. In

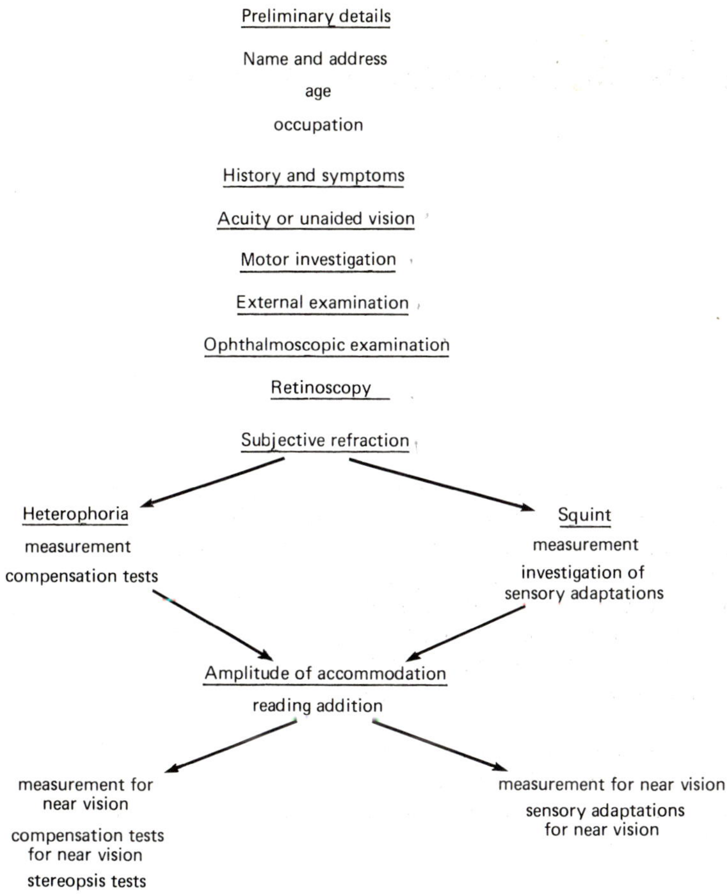

Figure 2.1. Summary of routine eye and vision examination

children, binocular anomalies can occur without any serious symptoms, due to the sensory adaptation. The onset of a squint at an early age is seldom accompanied by symptoms. However, a high percentage of patients will attend for examination because they are having symptoms which they associate with the eyes and vision, or come for a check because they have a history of binocular vision problems.

Headache is a common symptom. It may be caused by a very large variety of problems, many of which have nothing to do with the eyes or vision. It is important to determine if any headache is associated with the use of eyes. It is usual for decompensated heterophoria to cause some headache which occurs after prolonged use of the eyes, often under bad visual conditions. This type of headache is more likely to be in the frontal region of the head. Usually, headache due to binocular vision problems is less in intensity or absent in the morning after a night's sleep, and gets worse as the day wears on.

Diplopia is a less usual symptom in long-standing squint, as the sensory adaptation occurs. Its presence therefore indicates a deviation of recent onset. Such deviation may have a pathological cause, and therefore careful attention is given to the tests for comitancy. The patient may sometimes report that the double vision is greater in one direction of gaze. The patient should also be asked if the doubling is constant or intermittent, whether it is horizontal or vertical, and if it is associated with any particular use of the eyes. Incomitant deviations are more likely to have a vertical component. Double vision in heterophoria indicates that it is intermittently breaking down into a squint. This may be because the factors causing the decompensation have reached a serious state, but are still of a functional nature. Sometimes it is an early indication of an active pathological cause. In the latter case, the onset of intermittent diplopia is likely to be more sudden and dramatic.

Blurred vision is a very usual symptom in heterophoria. It can be associated with accommodative difficulties such as undercorrected presbyopia, or uncorrected hyperopia. In these cases, the blurred vision is more likely to be noticed by the patient during close work. Patients may also report general tiredness or soreness of the eyes or lids.

Poor stereopsis occurs with some binocular vision problems in which the patients report difficulty in judging distances.

If a squint is reported or is obvious to the practitioner, it is important to discover how long it has been present and if it is constant or intermittent. Where there is an hereditary factor or a history of orbital trauma during birth delivery, it is unlikely that squints will respond to non-operative treatment alone. It may be necessary to investigate the presence of history or symptoms which suggest other trauma or pathological conditions which contribute to the cause of the squint (see Chapter 16).

The family history may be important, as the presence of amblyopia or squint in a parent or near relative makes it more likely in the patient.

Another important part of the history is to gain an understanding of any previous treatment that may have been given. This may have included spectacles, occlusion, orthoptic exercises or an operation. In each case, it is necessary to discover the type of treatment given and the effect on the symptoms and the binocular condition. Generally, if a particular treatment has been tried and proved unsuccessful, it is not worth trying again.

The patient's general health may also be significant in binocular vision anomalies. Low general health may contribute to heterophoria becoming decompensated, and will make treatment more difficult.

Acuity or unaided vision

The unaided vision of each eye or the corrected acuity with the patient's own present glasses is usually measured with a standard Snellen letter chart. For young children, other kinds of apparatus may be more appropriate (see Chapter 15). If the patient does not wear a spectacle correction all the time, it is useful to record the vision with and without the correction, and to note any obvious effect on the binocular vision.

It is important to record the acuities early in the examination, as this often gives a clue to what may be expected in subsequent investigation. For example, an eye with reduced acuity is more likely to be the deviated eye.

In amblyopia, other details may be inferred from the way in which the patient reads the chart. Difficulty in reading the middle letters of a line in the correct order may suggest eccentric fixation with the small accompanying scotoma. This scotoma may show on the Amsler charts (see Chapter 11).

Motor investigation

The motor investigation will normally include:

(1) *Cover test* – which will indicate whether any deviation is a squint or heterophoria, the degree of deviation and some indication of compensation in heterophoria.
(2) *Motility test* – which investigates any restrictions of eye movements and the comitancy.
(3) *Associated reflexes* – which will include lid movements, convergence, the accommodative tests and pupil reflexes.

Cover test

This is largely an objective test relying on the critical observation of the practitioner. It is the only way to distinguish between heterophoria and squint, unless there is an obvious deviation which can be seen by looking at the patient. The cover test requires a lot of skill, but this can readily be acquired by practice. Essentially it consists of covering and uncovering each eye in turn, while the other eye fixes a letter on a distance chart or a suitable near fixation target.

As one eye is covered, the practitioner watches the other: any movement indicates that it was deviated, i.e. squinting, and had to move to take up fixation. As the cover is removed, the practitioner watches the eye which has been covered: any movement of this eye indicates that it was deviated under the cover and recovers when the cover is removed and it is free to take up fixation. In the absence of a squint, this shows heterophoria.

The test should be carried out for distance vision using a letter on the Snellen chart which can be easily read by the eye with the lowest acuity, but requires precise accommodation; it is repeated for near vision at the patient's usual working distance. It is useful to hold the occluder a few centimetres from the eye, so that while it occludes the eye from most of the visual field, the observer may peep round the edge and see the covered eye. However, it is important that most of the visual field is occluded, particularly from bright lights in the periphery which can stimulate abnormal movements in some patients. In performing the cover test, the eye is covered only for 1 or 2 seconds, so that the response to momentary dissociation is observed. The effect of longer dissociation can be observed by the alternating cover test method (see below).

COVER TEST IN SQUINT

This is illustrated in *Figure 2.2*, which shows the movements in right convergent squint, and in *Figure 2.3*, which shows right divergent squint with right hypertropia. The cover test will also help in investigating the other aspects of squint:

(1) *Constancy*. An intermittent squint may be present sometimes and binocular vision recovered at other times. Often this type of squint is not present until the cover test is performed, but the momentary dissociation is sufficient to make the squint manifest.

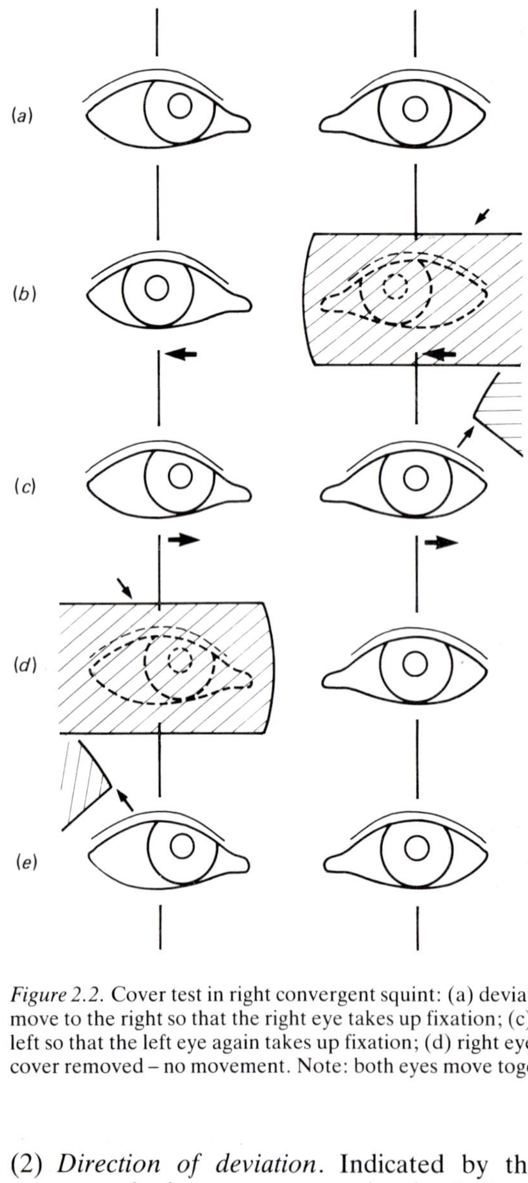

Figure 2.2. Cover test in right convergent squint: (a) deviated right eye; (b) left eye covered – both eyes move to the right so that the right eye takes up fixation; (c) left eye uncovered – both eyes move to the left so that the left eye again takes up fixation; (d) right eye covered – no movement of either eye; (e) cover removed – no movement. Note: both eyes move together in accordance with Hering's law

(2) *Direction of deviation.* Indicated by the direction of the movement; for example, in convergent squint the deviated eye will be seen to move outwards to take up fixation when the other eye is covered.
(3) *Eye preference.* In alternating squint, covering one eye will transfer the squint to the other eye which will continue to fix when the cover is removed. In such squints, a preference for fixation with one eye may be found; although fixation can be maintained with either eye, if the patient blinks or changes fixation momentarily, the fixation always reverts to the preferred eye. In other cases, the patient may be able to maintain fixation with either eye at will.
(4) *Degree of deviation.* With practice, the angle of the squint can be estimated from the amount of the movement. The degree may also be estimated by the

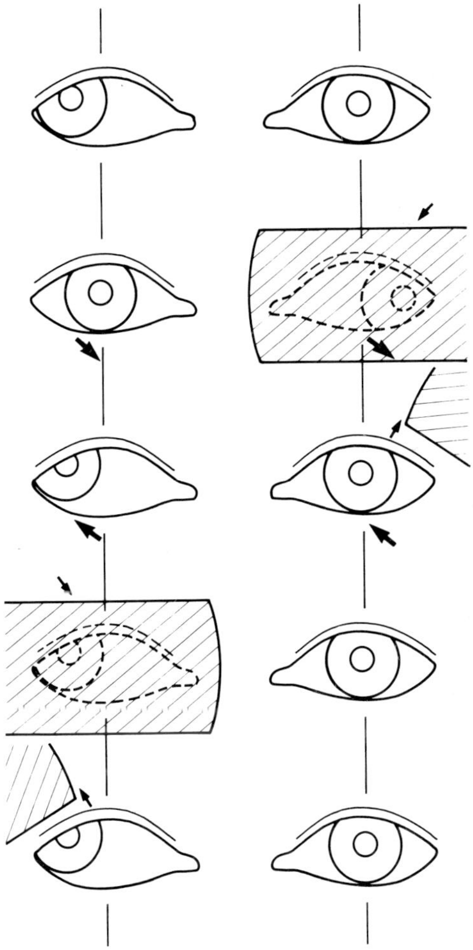

Figure 2.3. Cover test in right divergent squint with right hypertropia: (a) right eye deviated out and up; (b) left eye covered – both eyes move left and downwards so that the right eye takes up fixation; (c) left eye uncovered – both eyes move right and upwards so that the left eye again takes up fixation; (d) and (e) no movement of either eye as the squinting right eye is covered and uncovered

Hirschberg method (see *Figure 2.4*). It is now usual to measure angles of squint in prism dioptres. It must be noted that both these methods only give estimates which may be related to measurement taken by other means, see Prism measurement below.

COVER TEST IN HETEROPHORIA

This is illustrated with respect to esophoria in *Figure 2.5*. The eyes are straight until they are dissociated by covering one. Then the covered eye deviates into the heterophoric position behind the cover. It will be seen to make a recovery movement when the cover is removed. In the most simple cases (*Figure 2.5a–c*), the eye which is not covered will continue to fix without making any movements

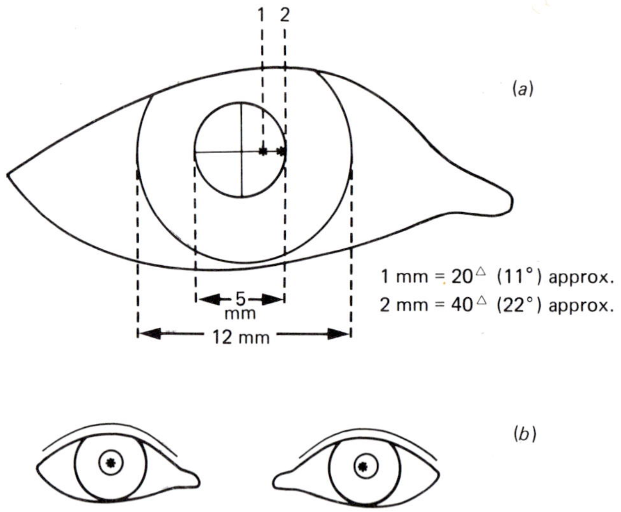

Figure 2.4. Hirschberg estimation method for the angle of squint. (a) The reflection of a light in the cornea appears displaced from the centre of the pupil by 1 mm for each 20^{Δ} (11°) of deviation of the eye. The position of the reflex relative to the pupil margin is shown for two deviations. (b) The appearance for a left divergent squint of about 20^{Δ}. This assumed that the angle kappa is zero, and the reflex is central in the right undeviated eye. In most hyperopes, kappa is 5^{Δ}–9^{Δ}, with the reflex on the nasal side of the pupil. In myopes, it is usually less, or central, or on the temporal side. The position of the reflex in the non-amblyopic eye (with the other eye covered) should be noted before the angle of squint is estimated binocularly by judging the difference in position of the reflex in the squinting eye. In a right convergent squint with a large angle kappa, the reflexes would therefore appear in the same positions as those shown in (b). (Angle kappa is the angular difference between the pupil centre and where the visual axis cuts the pupil plane)

either when the other is covered or when the cover is removed. However, it should be noted that this is not in accordance with Hering's law of equal eye movements.

Movements of both eyes may be seen on the removal of the cover in some cases (*Figure 2.5d–f*). This is particularly noticeable in large degrees of heterophoria. When the cover is removed, both eyes are seen to make a versional movement of about half the total phoria deviation; that is, they both move in the same direction, to the left or to the right. This versional movement is relatively quick, and is followed by a slower change of vergence of about the same magnitude. For the eye which has been covered, the second part of the recovery will be in the same direction as the versional movement. For the non-covered eye, the second movement will be a return to its fixation position. That is to say, the eye which is not covered will be seen to make an apparently irrelevant movement outwards (for esophoria) and back again to its fixation position. In the cases which show this pattern of movements, it will be noted that Hering's law does apply.

In heterophoria, the cover test movements are usually the same whether the left or the right eye is covered. In some cases, however, this is not so. In uncorrected anisometropes, the movement can be larger in one eye if a change in accommodation is required to keep the fixation target in focus when one eye is covered, but not when the other is covered.

In some patients, the versional pattern of movements may show when one eye is covered, but the simple pattern if the cover is applied to the other eye. These

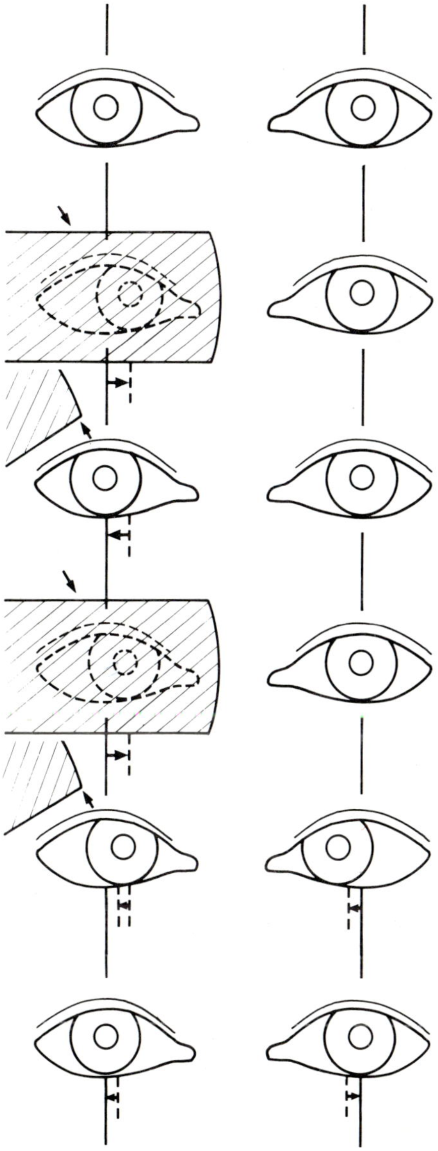

Figure 2.5. The cover test in esophoria. (a)–(c) From the 'straight' active position, the right eye moves inwards when dissociated by covering (b); it moves smoothly outwards to resume fixation with the other eye when the cover is removed (c). Note that the left (uncovered) eye does not move during the simple pattern of movements. (d)–(f) The 'versional pattern': the right eye moves inwards under the cover, as in the simple pattern (d); on removing the cover, both eyes move to the right by the same amount (about half the degree of the esophoria) (e); both eyes then diverge to the straight position (f)

patients have marked ocular dominance. The versional pattern is seen on removing the cover from the dominant eye: fixation is quickly transferred to the dominant eye by the versional movement, and the recovery from the heterophoric position occurs in the non-dominant eye. These patients often have slight amblyopia with a small central suppression area in the non-dominant eye, and are considered by some to be a variant of microtropia (see below).

The cover test helps in the investigation of heterophoria by giving information on the following:

(1) *Direction of deviation* – esophoria, exophoria, hyperphoria or cyclophoria.
(2) *Degree of deviation* – estimated from the amount of movement seen on removing the cover.
(3) *Factors affecting compensation* – assessed by observing the speed of the recovery movement. A smooth quick recovery movement usually indicates compensated heterophoria, but if it is a decompensated, the recovery is likely to be slow and hesitant.

COVER TEST IN MICROTROPIA

This may present different appearances. Squints with inconspicuously small angles exist, and have been described by a number of terms and as having various characteristics. These will be discussed in more detail in Chapter 13. Generally, microtropia is not detected with the cover test either because there is a small central scotoma of angular size no greater than the squint, or because there is abnormal retinal correspondence and eccentric fixation which both coincide in degree with the angle of the squint. In microtropia, therefore, the squinting eye is not seen to move to take up fixation when the dominant eye is covered as it would in other squints. However, in some cases of microtropia, the angle of the deviation may increase when one eye is covered. This may be seen as an apparent 'phoria movement' when the cover is removed. This movement may be particularly noticeable if the cover is held in place for a longer time, or if the alternating cover test (see below) is used. It may be assumed that in the active or habitual position, the eyes are held straighter under the influence of peripheral fusion. This condition was called 'monofixational phoria' (Parks and Eustis, 1961; see also Chapter 13).

OTHER COVER TEST OBSERVATIONS

Failure of an eye to take up fixation sometimes occurs in both squint and heterophoria. The experienced practitioner can see that an eye is deviated. The eye will move to take up fixation if the patient is asked to 'look very hard at' the fixation target, or is asked to look at a point a little higher than but close to the original fixation point; say 2 or 3 mm for near vision. The eye can then be seen to make a horizontal movement as well as the necessary very small vertical one.

There are several modifications to the cover test which will give further useful information in some cases.

ALTERNATING COVER TEST

When the cover test has been carried out as described above, it is sometimes useful to transfer the cover from one eye to the other and back several times. The degree of the deviation usually increases, making it easier to see. It also allows the full extent of the deviation to be appreciated.

Where no obvious squint was seen, it is useful to watch the eyes carefully to see if any recovery movement takes place when the cover is finally removed after the alternating cover test. This may give some indication of the degree of compensation, as poorly compensated heterophoria does not recover so readily or as smoothly after the alternating cover test.

PRISM MEASUREMENT

Measurement of the deviation can be carried out by placing a relieving prism before the eye to neutralize the cover test movement. This can be done using single prisms from a trial case, or more conveniently by the use of a prism bar (see *Figure 12.1*). The lowest power of prism that neutralizes the movement is taken as a measure of the deviation. This can be done in heterophoria or in squint.

In the case of a squint, the habitual angle is measured by taking the cover and the prism away from both eyes between changes of prism power. This allows the habitual angle to be retained during the prism measurement. The total angle can be measured by neutralizing the movement during the alternating cover test without removing the prism bar between movements of the cover. During prism measurements, irrelevant movement away from fixation and back again can make accuracy difficult. These can be minimized by holding the prism before the non-squinting eye, and observing the bilateral movement as the cover is removed.

It will also be noticed that when the correct relieving prism is in place, the corneal reflections of a fixation light appear symmetrically placed in the two eyes. Before applying the cover therefore, an estimate of angle can be made by increasing the prism power until the corneal reflections appear to be symmetrically placed. This is called the Krimsky test (Krimsky, 1943).

SUBJECTIVE COVER TEST ('PHI' TEST)

If there is a deviation, either heterophoria or squint, the patient will observe an apparent jump of the fixation point when the cover is transferred from one eye to the other. This apparent jump is known as 'phi' movement. In convergent deviations, the jump will appear to be against the movement of the cover; that is, if the cover is moved from the right eye *to the left*, the fixation point will appear to move to the *right*. A 'with' movement occurs in divergent deviations.

Latent nystagmus may also be revealed by the cover test. It shows as an oscillation of one or both eyes when one is covered (see Chapter 17).

VALUE OF COVER TEST

Although this section describing the cover test is quite lengthy, it will be appreciated that the cover test itself is a comparatively quick procedure, and a very great deal of useful information can be found in a few moments. Because it is so valuable as a diagnostic procedure and takes so little time, it should be incorporated in all routine eye examinations. The time taken to acquire the necessary skill in observation is well worth while.

Motility test

An examination of the binocular vision needs to explore the ability of the patient to move the eyes into all parts of the motor field. This is usually carried out by asking the patient to look at a pentorch light, which is moved in the motor field, while the patient is asked to follow it with the eyes, and keep the head still. This is usually done binocularly, and if there is any suspicion of abnormality, it is repeated monocularly with each eye. The binocular motor field is restricted by the patient's brow and nose to eye movements of about 25° from the primary position. This can be thought of as equivalent to holding the pentorch 50 cm from the patient's face and tracing out a square of approximately 50 cm. Inside this square, the patient can fix the light with both eyes. Beyond this, the light will be occluded from one eye by the nose or brow. It is useful, however, to move the light outside the square into the monocular fixation area, as this is similar to carrying out a cover test in peripheral directions of gaze. Latent deviations and incomitancies can sometimes be detected by doing this. If there is any doubt, an actual cover test can be carried out in the peripheral gaze position. The cover will eliminate peripheral fusion when this is done. A quick useful routine is as follows:

(1) *Fixation* is checked first, in each eye, by asking the patient to fix the pentorch with the eyes in the primary position, while the other eye is occluded. Each eye is observed to see that steady fixation is maintained, with no wandering. The position of the pentorch reflection in the cornea is also noted with respect to the pupil. It should be symmetrical between the two eyes; usually slightly nasal if the angle kappa is normal. Any asymmetry may indicate eccentric fixation (see Chapter 11).
(2) *Pursuit eye movements* as the light is moved horizontally across the field should be smooth with no jerks. Both eyes should follow the light evenly across the binocular motor field and out into the area of monocular fixation, first one way and then the other. The lid apertures should not vary appreciably as this is carried out. In crossed alternating fixation, a jump of both eyes can be seen as the patient changes fixation to the other eye on moving from one half of the motor field to the other (see Chapter 14, page 145).
(3) *Vertical movement of the eyes and lids* are checked by moving the pentorch slowly about 25 cm above the horizontal, and then 25 cm below. Both eyes should follow the movement with corresponding lid movements.
(4) *Comitancy* is next examined. This is done by moving the light across the upper part of the motor field to the right and then to the left. This includes the area of binocular fixation and the monocular part of the field. The patient is asked to say if any doubling occurs in the binocular area, and the practitioner observes any underaction or overshooting of one eye compared with the other. Incomitancy may be detected either by the subjective diplopia or by the practitioner's observation. The process is repeated across the lower part of the motor field (see Chapter 16).
(5) *Saccadic movements* are checked by asking the patient to change fixation from the pentorch held at the right of the field to the practitioner's finger held in the left of the field, pause and back to the pentorch. These movements should be smooth, quick and accurate.

The motility test is the only objective test for eye movements, but there are a number of subjective methods that can be used where there is diplopia. These may be useful in recently acquired deviations where suppression is unlikely, and they are described in Chapter 16, together with anomalies in ocular motility.

Associated reflexes

The third aspect of the motor investigation is concerned with the associated reflexes: convergence, accommodation and pupil reflexes. These constitute three synkinetic actions which normally come into play together during near vision. The oculomotor (third cranial) nerve serves all of these, so that disturbances of one may be accompanied by the others (see Chapter 16 for pathological causes of recent onset).

CONVERGENCE

There are two aspects of convergence movements. The first is concerned with pursuit convergence: following an object brought slowly closer to the eyes by converging to retain a foveal image in both eyes. The second convergence movement concerns changing fixation from one object to another at a different distance: a re-fixation task for which there is the added stimulus of physiological diplopia. This second convergence movement will be referred to as 'jump convergence'. The investigation of convergence should include both pursuit and jump convergence.

Near point of convergence

This is used as a measure of pursuit convergence. A suitable target is brought slowly towards the eyes from a distance of about 50 cm and on the median line until the patient reports that it doubles and/or the practitioner sees that one eye has ceased to converge. The patient should wear reading glasses where appropriate. With most older patients, the near point of convergence will be closer to the eyes than the near point of accommodation, and the target will be seen to blur before it doubles. The convergence should still be investigated even if the target is blurred.

Jump convergence test

The patient is asked to fix a small object placed at about 50 cm from the eyes, and then to change fixation to a second object introduced at 15 cm. The patient's eyes should be seen to converge promptly and smoothly from the more distant object to the nearer one. Version movement of both eyes, hesitant or slow convergence, or no movement, are all abnormal (Pickwell and Hampshire, 1981).

The assessment of convergence by clinical tests needs to indicate if it will be adequate to cope with the needs of the patient in near vision. This can be decided by considering both convergence tests together; a near point of convergence between 10 and 15 cm and good jump convergence are taken as adequate. A fuller discussion of convergence anomalies is included in Chapter 6 under 'Convergence insufficiency'.

ACCOMMODATION

The amplitude of accommodation is the measure by which the eyes can change focus; it is the range from the far point to the near point in dioptres. Because it is measured from the far point, the measurement needs to be taken with the distance correction in place. It is therefore assessed after the refractive part of the routine examination.

The usual clinical method is to ask the patient to look at small print on a card which is moved slowly towards the eye until the patient reports that clear vision cannot be maintained. The card is mounted on a near-point rule so that the dioptral distance can be read from the rule. In the case of a young patient with a near point close to the eyes, a negative sphere (−4.00 DS) is held before the eyes so that the accommodative range is moved to the middle of the rule (DS = dioptres of spherical power). The value of this sphere is then added to the reading. This is a subjective method and its accuracy depends on the patient's ability to distinguish a blur point, on the depth of focus and other variables, but is a standard clinical procedure.

TABLE 2.1. Variation of minimum amplitude of accommodation with age: Emsley's figures (after Duane) and quoted by Giles (1960) for monocular measurements

Age (yr)	10	15	20	25	30	35	40	45	50	60	70
Ocular accommodation (D)	11.0	10.25	9.5	8.5	7.5	6.5	5.5	3.5	2.0	1.25	1.0

The amplitude of accommodation decreases with age between 10 and 65 years. Mean values have been given by a number of authorities of which Duane is the most widely accepted (Duane, 1912). In practice, it is the minimum value of the spread of amplitudes for normal individuals in any age group that is clinically important. Such values are quoted from Giles (1960) in *Table 2.1*. These are for the European races living in temperate climates. It is accepted that there is a racial variation or differences caused by geographical area of upbringing (Duke-Elder, 1970) which give a lower amplitude. Otherwise, an amplitude lower than the value in *Table 2.1* is suspicious. Abnormalities of accommodation related to binocular vision are considered in later chapters.

PUPIL REFLEXES

Anomalies of pupil reflexes may also help in the diagnosis of binocular difficulties due to neural disturbances. It is necessary therefore to check the pupil reflexes to light, and in near vision. The direct light reflex is checked by shining a light into one eye and observing the pupil constriction. At the same time, the consensual reflex is checked by observing the constriction of the pupil of the other eye. This is repeated by shining the light into the other eye. The near-vision pupil reflex is checked by asking the patient to look at a distance object and then at one about 25 cm from the eyes: the pupil constriction accompanying the accommodation and convergence is observed.

When checking the pupil reflexes, abnormalities in size, irregularities in shape or inequalities between the right and left pupils should be noted.

External and ophthalmoscopic examinations

During the early part of the examinations, general observation of the patient can take place. With respect to binocular vision it is appropriate to notice:

(1) Compensatory head postures that may be adopted in incomitant deviations – a head-tilt, a rotation of the face to the left or right, or the face turned up or down.
(2) Any obvious squint.
(3) Exophthalmos – protrusion of one or both eyes.
(4) Epicanthus – a fold of skin across the inner angle of the lids seen in some European children, and frequently in oriental races, which may give the appearance of a convergent squint; the cover test should confirm whether a squint is actually present.
(5) Anatomical asymmetries, malformations or signs of injury.
(6) Ptosis or other anomalies of the lid openings.
(7) Scleral signs of previous squint operations, which may show as a scar or a local reddening.

It is essential that an ophthalmoscopic examination be carried out to discover any signs of active pathology, before proceeding to treat a functional deviation.

Retinoscopy and subjective refraction

In very many binocular vision anomalies, the correction of the refractive error is important in the treatment. For example, in many heterophoria cases no other treatment is required, and in accommodative squint it can be the principal treatment. Exact and full determination of the refractive error is therefore essential. The function of the refractive correction in particular anomalies is described in later chapters, and it is not the function of this book to give details of different methods of refraction. However, it must be emphasized that great care must be taken to ensure that each eye is given the correction that will provide a sharp retinal image. This correction should be balanced between the two eyes in the sense that it is equally clear without either eye accommodating. This can be done objectively by passing the retinoscope light quickly from one eye to the other to ensure that, at the conclusion of the retinoscopic examination, both eyes are neutralized simultaneously. In heterophoria where there is binocular fixation, this is best done by asking the patient to fix the retinoscope once the monocular error has been neutralized with distance fixation (Barrett, 1945; Hodd, 1951). Balancing can be carried out subjectively by an infinity balance or septum method (Turville, 1946), by a projected polaroid vectograph method (Grolman, 1966), or by an equalizing technique using alternative occlusion or a fogging method (Borish, 1970).

In squint or amblyopia, the retinoscopy is more important, as an accurate subjective test may not be possible on the amblyopic eye. Extra care must be taken to ensure that refraction is on the visual axis. In divergent or larger angle convergent squints, the practitioner can move round in line with the visual axis. The correct position can be judged by centring the reflection in the cornea of the retinoscope light. In the case of cycloplegic refraction, the patient can be asked to look at the retinoscope and the other eye occluded.

Measurement and assessment of deviation

In heterophoria, the first requirement is to assess if it is compensated or not when the correction is in place. If it was not compensated before the spectacle correction was found, but it is now better compensated, the correction is indicated as a part of the management of the heterophoria and in alleviating the symptoms. Assessing the degree of compensation with and without the spectacles is discussed in Chapter 3. The assessment should be made for distance or for near vision, according to when the symptoms occur. The measurement of the degree of heterophoria and investigation of stereopsis may be required as part of the assessment.

In squint, the angle of deviation is measured for distance and for near vision with the refractive correction in place, so that its effect on the angle can be determined. The measurement can be made with the cover test, as described above. In the case of long-standing squint, binocular sensory adaptations may have developed to alleviate diplopia and confusion. The extent and nature of these adaptations will need to be determined. Sensory adaptation and their investigation is covered in the chapters on squint, but a routine is summarized here:

(1) Retinal correspondence can be investigated with Bagolini striate lenses. The depth of abnormal retinal correspondence can be assessed with a filter bar before the deviated eye until diplopia or suppression occurs.

(2) Suppression can be investigated by the ease with which the patient gets diplopia, and the depth of suppression determined with a filter bar before the undeviated eye until diplopia occurs.
(3) Physiological diplopia may be elicited at a distance where the visual axes cross; this can indicate a good prognosis.

References

BARRETT, C. D. (1945). Sources of error and working methods in retinoscopy. *British Journal of Physiological Optics*, **5,** 35–40

BORISH, J. M. (1970). *Clinical Refraction*, 3rd edn. Professional Press, Chicago, pp. 752–755

DUANE, A. (1912). Normal values of accommodation at all ages. *Transactions of the Section on Ophthalmology of the American Medical Association,* pp. 383–391

DUKE-ELDER, SIR STEWART (1970). *System of Ophthalmology*, vol. V. *Ophthalmic Optics and Refraction*. Kimpton, London, p. 459

GILES, G. H. (1960). *The Principles and Practice of Refraction*. Hammond & Hammond, London, p. 193

GROLMAN, B. (1966). Binocular refraction: a new system. *New England Optometrist*, **17**(6), 118–123

HODD, F. A. B. (1951). The measurement of spherical refraction by retinoscopy. *Transactions of the International Congress of the British Optical Association*, pp. 191–291

KRIMSKY, E. (1943). The binocular examination of the young child. *American Journal of Ophthalmology,* **26,** 624

PARKS, M. M. and EUSTIS, A. T. (1961). Monofixational phoria. *American Orthoptic Journal*, **11,** 38–42

PICKWELL, L. D. and HAMPSHIRE, R. (1981). The significance of inadequate convergence. *Ophthalmic Physiological Optics*, **1**(1), 13–18

TURVILLE, A. E. (1946). *Outline of Infinity Balance*. Raphael, London

Part II

Heterophoria

3

Evaluation of heterophoria

The purpose of evaluating the heterophoria is to determine if it is decompensated; giving rise to symptoms or to suppression. If it is decompensated, the evaluation should identify what factors are causing it to have become so. In general, it is heterophoria that has been fully compensated but becomes decompensated that gives rise to symptoms. The factors that cause heterophoria to become decompensated are discussed in Chapter 1 under the heading Compensation. If these factors can be identified, the management will consist of removing or relieving as many of them as possible.

The routine examination of the eyes and vision includes the investigation of heterophoria, and the information revealed must then be evaluated; that is, the results from all the parts of the examination are considered together, to discover the significance of each part and what it all adds up to in total. It may be found that it fits a recognizable pattern, which is called the diagnosis. On the basis of this conclusion, a decision can be reached on what to do for the patient – the management of the case. This process can be summarized as follows:

Investigation + Evaluation = Diagnosis → Management

This formula represents the general principle of clinical procedure; the results of the examination are evaluated to reach a diagnosis. Then experience may suggest the best way of dealing with the particular condition that has been diagnosed.

As previously mentioned, some heterophoria can be a secondary effect of an active disease or pathological process or from recent injury. This type will be called 'pathological' heterophoria. It is usually incomitant, i.e. varies with the direction of gaze. In some directions of gaze it may even break down into a squint and double vision occurs. As already explained (see Chapter 2), some parts of the routine examination are particularly important in the detection of pathological deviations, and these assume more significance in the total evaluation when such a diagnosis is reached. These aspects are dealt with more fully in Chapter 16. At this stage, the emphasis is on comitant (non-pathological) heterophoria, and it may be assumed that there is no pathological element unless otherwise stated.

As most people have some degree of heterophoria, it is obviously important to decide in which cases it is likely to give rise to troubles. That is to say, it is necessary to distinguish the compensated from the decompensated heterophoria. If the heterophoria is compensated, there is no need to evaluate it further. If it is decompensated, further evaluation is required to see which of the classifications describes the appearance presented with a particular patient.

In deciding if heterophoria is compensated, the results of all parts of the routine examination need to be considered, but some sections or tests are particularly important. Sometimes the routine eye examination may also suggest that some supplementary tests should be carried out to help in the evaluation. The following parts of the routine or supplementary tests are particularly useful in assessing heterophoria:

(1) Symptoms.
(2) Cover test.
(3) Refraction.
(4) Measurement of the degree of heterophoria.
(5) Prism vergences.
(6) Partial dissociation tests.
(7) Fixation disparity tests.
(8) Suppression tests.
(9) Stereoscopic tests.
(10) Binocular acuity.

Symptoms

Symptoms will usually be present in decompensated heterophoria. Less usually, suppression develops to such a stage that symptoms are not present. However, there is no set of symptoms that is characteristic of heterophoria, so it can be inferred that it is the main cause of the trouble. The symptoms that accompany decompensated heterophoria are largely those which may be present in many other difficulties. It can, however, be said that where there are no symptoms and no suppression, any heterophoria is compensated. When symptoms are present, the practitioner must decide if these are due to the heterophoria or to some other cause. It is only by considering the symptoms together with the other findings that the total picture enables the diagnosis of phoria trouble to be made.

In general, the symptoms resulting from decompensated heterophoria can be associated with some particular use of the eyes for prolonged periods, and these symptoms are lessened or alleviated by resting the eyes. It follows that, in general, the symptoms will be less in the morning and increase during the day. In heterophoria, they are more frequently associated with near visual tasks.

Decompensated heterophoria can give rise to the following symptoms:

(1) *Headache.* Usually, this in the frontal regions of the head, but can be occipital.
(2) *Aching eyes.* The patient says that the eyes hurt after a lot of close work, or that there is pain 'behind the eyes'. In heterophoria, this is usually a dull pain, and is therefore described by the patient as an ache. It usually follows a long period of intensive use of the eyes for reading, sewing, television, cinema, etc.
(3) *Diplopia.* In heterophoria this is intermittent, and is worse after prolonged use of the eyes for a particular task. The diplopia that accompanies a pathological deviation is usually more sudden in onset, and seldom associated with any particular use of the eyes for lengthy periods.
(4) *Blurred vision.* Uncorrected refractive error may put a stress on the accommodation–convergence relationship, which results in decompensated

heterophoria. Conversely in, other cases, where there is no refractive error, high degrees of phoria can induce excessive accommodative effort and blurred vision results. Blurred near vision is the symptom most often present, particularly in older patients. It is usually associated with the need for an adequate reading addition. Decompensated heterophoria may also be present and sometimes requires attention even when the reading glasses have been given. If the symptoms are still present, the heterophoria needs re-evaluation.

(5) *Accommodative difficulties.* Patients may report that distance vision is blurred immediately following prolonged periods of close work.
(6) *Stereopsis problems.* Sometimes there are difficulties in depth perception reported by the patient; e.g. in ball games, pouring liquids into receptacles.
(7) *Monocular comfort.* Sometimes a patient notices that vision is more comfortable if one eye is closed. This can also be due to photophobia, but also seems to be associated with heterophoria problems.
(8) *Sore eyes.* The patient may describe a feeling of soreness or the lid margins may be inflamed.
(9) *General irritation.* The difficulty in maintaining comfortable single vision may result in the patient reporting a feeling of agitation or of nervous exhaustion.

Cover test

The method of performing the cover test is described in Chapter 2. Here, we are concerned with evaluating the results. In heterophoria cases, three things should be noted during the cover test:

(1) *Direction of recovery.* The direction of the recovery movement will indicate how the eye was deviated under the cover before its removal. For distance fixation, most patients show little or no movement. For near fixation, the average patient becomes gradually more exophoric from the mid-twenties and has about 6^{Δ} of physiological exophoria by the age of 65 years (Pickwell and Freier, 1983). Obvious departures from this usual state may be decompensated, depending on the other factors.
(2) *Degree of phoria.* The larger the amount of heterophoria present, the more likely it is to be decompensated. However, quite small departures from the normal degree are sometimes decompensated, and sometimes high degrees are compensated.
(3) *Quality of recovery.* The speed and ease of recovery are also a good guide to the degree of compensation. A quick, smooth recovery is likely to indicate compensated heterophoria, whereas a slow, hesitant or jerking recovery movement usually accompanies decompensation.

It will be seen that all three of the above aspects of the recovery movement to the cover test need to be considered in deciding if the heterophoria is compensated.

Refraction

Because of the accommodation–convergence relationship, there is an association between esophoria and uncorrected hyperopia in young patients. When the patient is able to accommodate to compensate for the hyperopia and thereby achieve clear vision, the extra accommodation brought into play will induce extra convergence effort. Usually this will show as esophoria and there will be an unusual stress on the binocular vision; the esophoria may be decompensated. This will be exaggerated in near vision when the amount of accommodation required may be a large proportion of the patient's total amplitude. In such cases, the degree of the heterophoria is usually less with the refractive correction, and the clinical signs of decompensation will be less apparent. In hyperopic cases with exophoria, the correction may make the decompensation worse.

In myopia, the link with exophoria is not so marked, but the refractive correction usually assists the compensation.

The effect of the refractive correction on the heterophoria should always be noted.

Although there are methods of binocular refraction which do not require the use of an occluder, such as the Humphriss immediate contrast method (Humphriss and Woodruff, 1962), most refractive methods occlude each eye in turn. Binocular vision is suspended for a short time, while each eye is tested separately. When both the monocular refractions have been completed, the occluder is removed and the eyes are free to resume binocular vision. In compensated heterophoria, this is done promptly and the binocular acuity is found to be slightly better by several letters on the best line of the Snellen chart. The patient will usually report a slight subjective improvement if asked.

The removal of the occluder may therefore be regarded as an important part of the assessment of compensation. The patient is asked to look at the best line of Snellen letters which was seen monocularly, the occluder is removed, and the patient is asked if it is better or worse. In most cases, it will be better, and the binocular acuity can be recorded. Where there are binocular vision problems, the patient may report that the appearance is not quite so good, or may hesitate and blink a few times before comfortable binocular vision is restored. In some cases diplopia may be reported, and the patient may have to make a convergent movement to look at a near object before binocular vision can be obtained. Sometimes the binocular acuity may be slightly worse than that of each eye monocularly. All these reactions indicate binocular vision difficulty, and suggest decompensated heterophoria. Attention to the proper procedure in removing the occluder requires little time, but can give valuable information about compensation. Where binocular difficulties are suggested at this stage, particular attention to this aspect is indicated in the rest of the routine examination.

Measurement of degree of heterophoria

It was previously assumed that higher degrees of heterophoria were more likely to be decompensated than lower degrees. The degree of dissociated heterophoria was therefore routinely measured. However, it has long been recognized that high degrees of heterophoria are often compensated and low degrees decompensated. Recent work has failed to show any relationship between the degree of the heterophoria and either the presence of symptoms or decompensation by other tests (Yekta, Jenkins and Pickwell, 1987). It is clear that there is no justification for measuring heterophoria routinely. Indeed, the time is much better spent on other procedures.

In accommodative deviations, a hyperopic correction does reduce the degree of heterophoria in the short term. Measurement in these cases may give an indication of the likely effect of wearing the glasses. If the heterophoria is reduced by the glasses, it is likely that it will become compensated by wearing the glasses without any other treatment. However, other tests for compensation may give similar indications.

There is no evidence to show that other non-surgical treatments reduce the degree of heterophoria even when it relieves the symptoms and restores compensation. The degree of heterophoria cannot therefore be used as a monitor of the progress of treatment.

The measurement may be carried out for 6 m and for the reading distance. For example, this can be done by the Maddox rod (or multiple groove) method. The Maddox groove consists of a series of very high power cylindrical elements which blur a spot of light into a streak. When placed before one eye, the Maddox groove produces this streak, which cannot be fused with the spot seen with the other eye at the same time. The eyes are therefore dissociated and take up the heterophoria position. The amount of the deviation can be noted by the patient subjectively as the separation of the spot and streak judged by a tangent scale, or by the power of the prism required to restore the streak to the central position where it appears to pass through the spot. In other methods, the eyes are dissociated by a plano prism, introduced so that the images of the two eyes are separated in one meridian and fusion is prevented. The deviation of the eyes can be measured by the displacement of the two images in the other meridian.

For near vision, the same sorts of method may be used, or the phoria measurement made with a Maddox wing test. This employs a number of septa to dissociate one part of the field from that seen by the other eye. The measurement is read by the patient where an arrow seen by one eye points to a tangent scale seen by the other.

Most subjective methods of measuring heterophoria have limitations which make them unreliable on some patients. The degree of dissociation and the stimulus to accommodation may vary. The measurement obtained with these methods should be taken, at best, only as another factor in helping to evaluate the heterophoria. Although they are time-honoured procedures, it is doubtful if they are the best way of spending time in a routine examination.

Prism vergences

The prism vergence tests assess the amount of prism which can be introduced before the eyes before fusion breaks down and blurred or double vision occurs. These are sometimes referred to as 'fusional reserves', or as 'binocular duction measurements'. They may be measured with rotary or variable prism devices or with a prism bar. The patient is asked to look at letters which are small enough to require precise fixation and accommodation. The prism power is introduced and slowly increased until the patient reports that the print is blurring or doubling. The prism is then reduced until clear single vision is recovered. The prism power at which these occur is noted, and recorded as the prism vergence to 'blur point' (the relative convergence), to break point and to recovery point. This may be carried out with prism base-in (divergent amplitude or negative fusional reserve), with prism base-out (convergent amplitude or positive fusional reserve), or with vertical prism (vertical amplitude). Measurements are taken for distance and for near vision. It is better to measure the base-in vergence before the base-out, as the exercising of excessive convergence tends to decrease the divergence and produce false results.

A number of criteria have been suggested for the assessment of prism vergences. Sheard (1930) suggested that the opposing prism vergence to the blur point should be at least twice the degree of the phoria. This seems to apply to exophoria at distance vision as a good working rule. Earlier, Percival (1892) had proposed that, for comfort, the working fixation point should lie in the middle third of the total amplitude obtained by adding the base-in vergence to the base-out. That is to say, the opposing prism vergences should be balanced within the limits that one should not be less than half the other. This rule seems to be appropriate for near vision only. *Table 3.1* shows the mean values for a number of normal persons (Pickwell, 1965); this seems to agree with other sample values (Davis, 1937; Morgan, 1944). It will be noted that Percival's middle third rule does not apply to these values for distance vision.

TABLE 3.1. Average values of prism vergence: horizontally for distance and near vision; vertically they are same for distance and near

	Prism vergences (Δ)		
	To blur	*To break*	*To recovery*
Distance vision (6 m)			
base-in vergence	–	5–9	4
base-out vergence	7–10	15–23	8–12
Near vision (33–40 cm)			
base-in vergence	11–15	18–24	7–15
base-out vergence	14–20	18–24	7–15
Vertical prism vergences			
right superduction (base-down R.E.)	2–4 } balanced*		
right infraction (base-up R.E.)	2–4 } balanced*		

*It is more important that the vertical measurements should be nearly the same, than that they should be high.

It should also be noted that the base-in vergence for distance is very small in comparison with other values, and that there is seldom any blur when measuring the divergence amplitude for distance vision. Perhaps the most significant aspect of this particular measurement is when it becomes excessively large, e.g. over 9^{Δ}, to break. This seems to indicate divergence excess (see Chapter 6).

Partial dissociation tests

Methods for measuring the degree of heterophoria require complete dissociation of the two eyes, e.g. the Maddox groove or the wing test. Another approach is to dissociate only part of the visual field by placing an impediment of a controlled extent in the way of binocular vision and to see what disturbance this causes. These methods leave part of the visual field common to both eyes, which provides a stimulus to fusion. The term used to describe this is 'fusion lock': it may be the central fixation area or it can be a peripheral fusion lock. The dissociation is achieved either by a septum or by a method of cross-polarization. Several

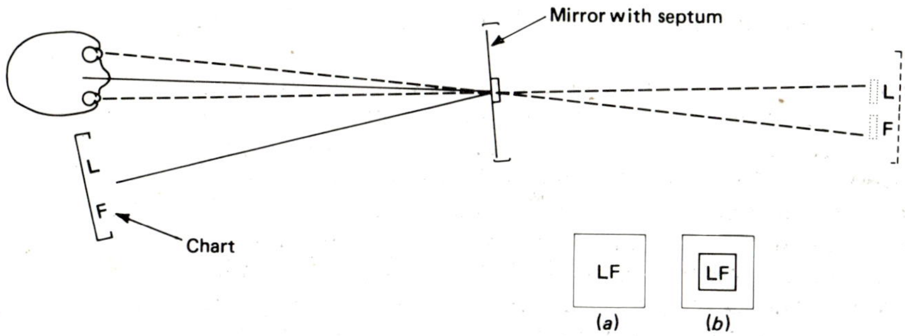

Figure 3.1. Infinity balance – general principle. A chart containing the letters L and F is seen reflected in the mirror. A septum in the centre of the mirror occludes the letter L from the right eye and the letter F from the left, so that the patient has partial dissociation of the field. F is seen with the right eye only, and L with the left only. The surrounding chart can be seen with both eyes, and its stimulus to stable binocular vision can be strengthened by a black frame (or 'binocular lock') seen with both eyes round the septum (b). A chart without the fusion lock (a) is also shown

suggestions have been made to provide a variable amount of dissociation, so that the amount which just causes a breakdown in binocular vision can be measured. This can be done by varying the width of a septum as in the Esdaile–Turville equilibrium test of 1927, or its position as in the Mitchell (1953) stability test; neither of these are now in common use. Suggestions for variable aperture which would allow a central lock have also been made – the Bishop–Harman diaphragm test of 1910 for near vision, and the Aldersley aperture test of 1936 for distance.

Turville's infinity balance (TIB) method has been widely used in Britain since its introduction (Turville, 1946), and has led to polarization methods for projection charts used in America (Morgan, 1960).

In the TIB or septum test, the septum dissociates the central parts of the binocular field, leaving the periphery with undisturbed binocular vision (see *Figure 3.1*). This allows binocular balancing of the refractive correction, as described below. In compensated heterophoria the eyes maintain their normal positions, but the degree of dissociation has been chosen so that, in decompensated phoria, a slight deviation occurs. The patient can see this as an abnormal position of the central areas – F and L in the infinity balance test. This may be horizontal or vertical, and the degree of compensation can be estimated by finding the smallest prism which will restore the central dissociated parts of the field to their normal positions. This prism will be less than an actual measurement of the phoria. This approach is particularly useful in hyperphoria.

Experience has shown that decompensation can sometimes be caused by an unbalanced spectacle correction, and the infinity balance allows this to be checked first. Binocular balance for near vision can also be checked by tests incorporated in most modern near-vision test units (Mallett, 1966b; 1966c). Where vision with one eye appears slightly clearer for distance or for near, the effect of adding +0.25 DS first before the eye with less clear image is tried. If this does not equalize, it is tried before the clearer eye to see if this will balance the acuities without blurring the clearer eye. If there is still inequality, a −0.25 DS is tried before the eye with the less clear image. When such a small addition produces equally clear images, it is incorporated in the prescription (*Figure 3.2*).

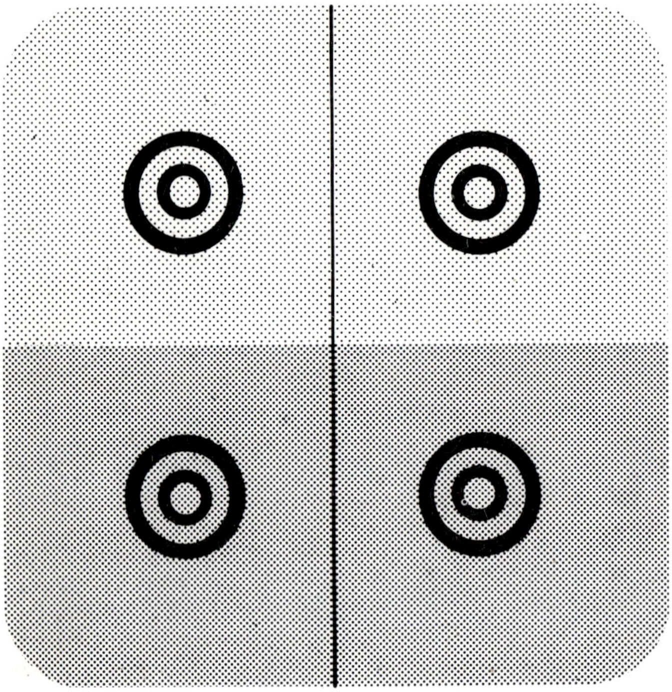

Figure 3.2. The binocular bichromatic test: this is used with a septum on the mirror to dissociate the right and left halves of the chart, so that one target is seen on a red and one on a green background with each eye. A bichromatic spherical balance can be made for the right eye at the same times as for the left, even if the acuities are not quite equal

It will also be appreciated that when the central parts (monocular) of the field appear to the patient to be displaced, the peripheral (binocular) field is not seen double. This is usually considered to be a fixation disparity effect.

Fixation disparity tests

In normal binocular vision, the fovea of one eye corresponds with a small area centred on the fovea of the other eye – Panum's area. Similarly every other point on the retina of one eye corresponds with a small area in the other eye. This point-to-area correspondence means that if a deviation of one eye starts to occur, no diplopia will be seen until the eye has deviated enough to move the image out of Panum's area. The eyes can therefore be deviated by a very small amount, which is less than 0.25^{Δ}, before any doubling is noticed. This very small deviation from fixation without diplopia is called 'fixation disparity'. It is very likely to occur when binocular vision is under stress; that is, in decompensated heterophoria. Tests which detect fixation disparity are therefore very useful in assessing decompensation. The deviation can occur in one eye or in both eyes, but because the magnitude is so small it cannot be seen with the cover test. Although fixation disparity has been detected objectively with special ophthalmoscopic methods (Pickwell and Stockley, 1960), all clinical tests are subjective.

Smc

The Mallett fixation disparity unit is such a test designed to detect the fixation disparity that is most likely to occur when there is decompensated heterophoria. Apparatus is designed for use at distance (Mallett, 1966a) and also for near vision (Mallett, 1964). In both tests, there is a central fixation target, the word OXO, seen with both eyes, and two monocular marks in line with the X, one seen with each eye (see *Figure 3.3*). Dissociation of the monocular marks is obtained by cross-polaroid filters. In fixation disparity, the images will be displaced slightly on the retina. Having no corresponding image in the same place on the other retina, the monocular markers will be given a visual direction associated with the retinal area stimulated, while the binocular image OXO, will be seen centrally. The monocular markers will therefore appear to the patient to be displaced from their alignment with the X.

The Mallett units do not measure the degree of the fixation disparity; that is, the amount by which the eye is actually deviated. This can, however, be estimated by the degree of the apparent misalignment compared with the letters OXO. What can be measured is the degree of prism relief required to neutralize the fixation disparity and restore the monocular markers to alignment with the X. This is called the 'associated phoria', and is distinguished from the 'dissociated phoria' which is revealed by methods which give complete dissociation such as the cover test, Maddox groove, etc. The angle of the actual fixation disparity is correlated with the magnitude of the associated phoria. Where the apparent degree of fixation disparity is high and the associated phoria is several prism dioptres, the possibility of decompensated heterophoria is very likely. Experience shows that some patients have small amounts of fixation disparity, but there is no other reason to suspect decompensation. It is therefore assumed that some fixation disparity must be physiological and a theory proposing that it is a purposeful error in the eyes' alignment which is a part of the convergence mechanism has some supporting evidence (Schor, 1979). Fixation disparity, however, increases when under prism stress, and it has also been shown to increase under the stress of working in inadequate illumination (Pickwell, Yekta and Jenkins, 1987), working at too close a reading distance (Pickwell, Jenkins and Yekta, 1987), and at the end of a day's close work (Yekta, Jenkins and Pickwell, 1987). As it may be either physiological or the result of binocular stress, the presence of fixation disparity suggests decompensation of the heterophoria which needs to be confirmed by other factors: the presence of symptoms; foveal suppression areas; anomalies in stereopsis or reduced binocular acuity compared with monocular; (see below).

The Mallett near-vision fixation disparity unit also incorporates tests for suppression in the foveal area, near acuity and for stereoscopic vision. As we have seen these are important in assessing the decompensation (Mallet, 1979). The Mallett units are also very useful in prescribing prism and other modifications to the spectacle prescription (see Chapter 4). These units have been designed and modified in the light of clinical experience and experimental findings, and they provide very useful methods of assessing the compensation.

It will be appreciated that, as the degree of fixation disparity can be changed by prisms, it is possible to plot the degree of fixation disparity against the power of the prism (Ogle, 1950). Several types of curve have been found, of which Type I is the most frequent and is illustrated in *Figure 3.4(a)*. Fixation disparity (in minutes of arc) is plotted vertically (y-axis) against the prism power (in prism dioptres) horizontally (x-axis). It will be noticed that the middle part of this typical sigma-shaped curve has a flatter slope; fixation disparity changes less over the

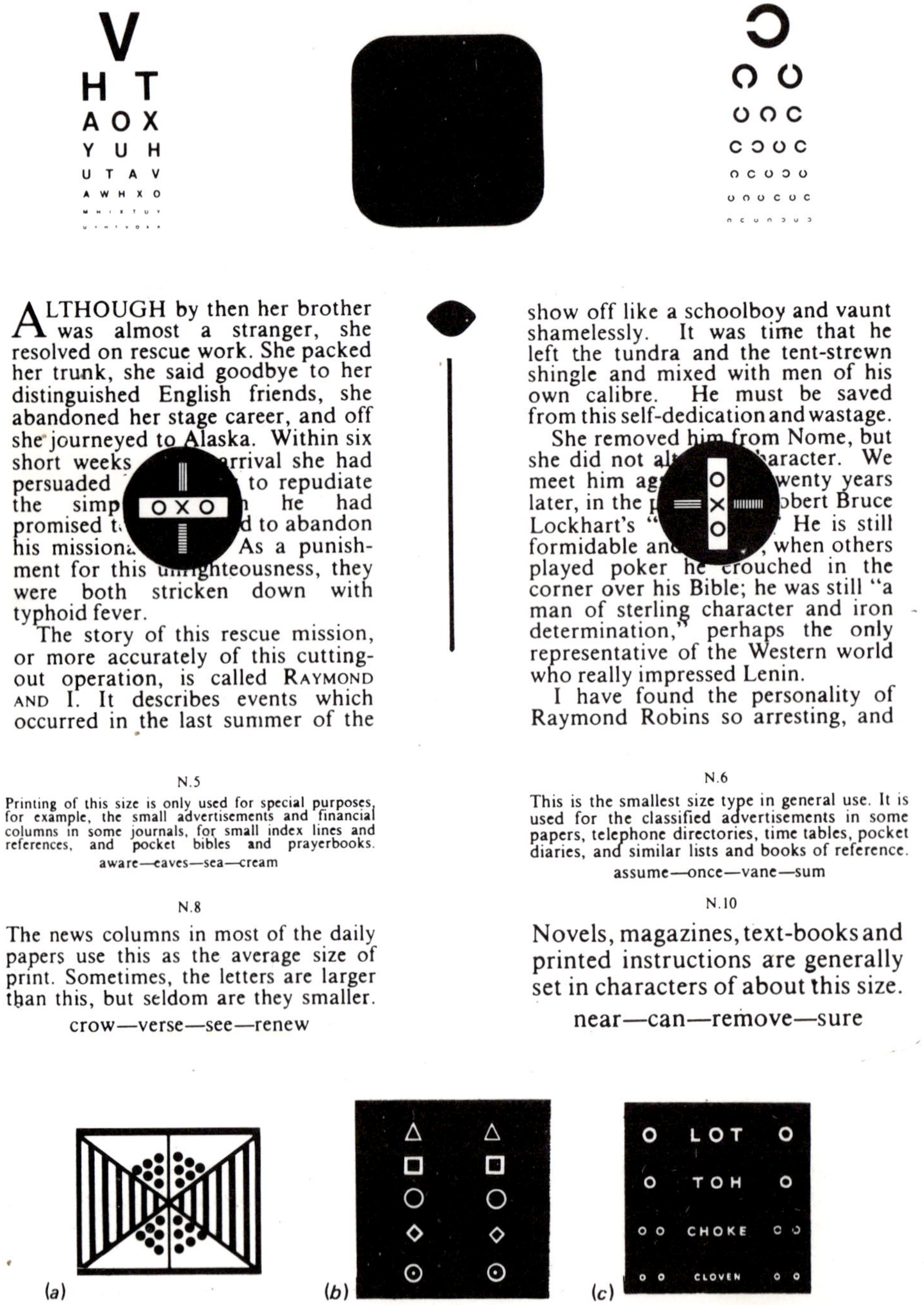

Figure 3.3 Mallett near-vision fixation disparity test: in black circles superimposed on printed passages, horizontal on left and vertical on the right. The letters OXO are seen binocularly, and the rectangular bars are cross-polarized to be seen one with each eye. The patient is asked to undertake the normal near-visual task of reading before the fixation disparity testing. The three inset figures below can be rotated in turn in the top black aperture of the test: (a) polarized bichromatic balance test, (b) stereoscopic vision chart, (c) suppression chart

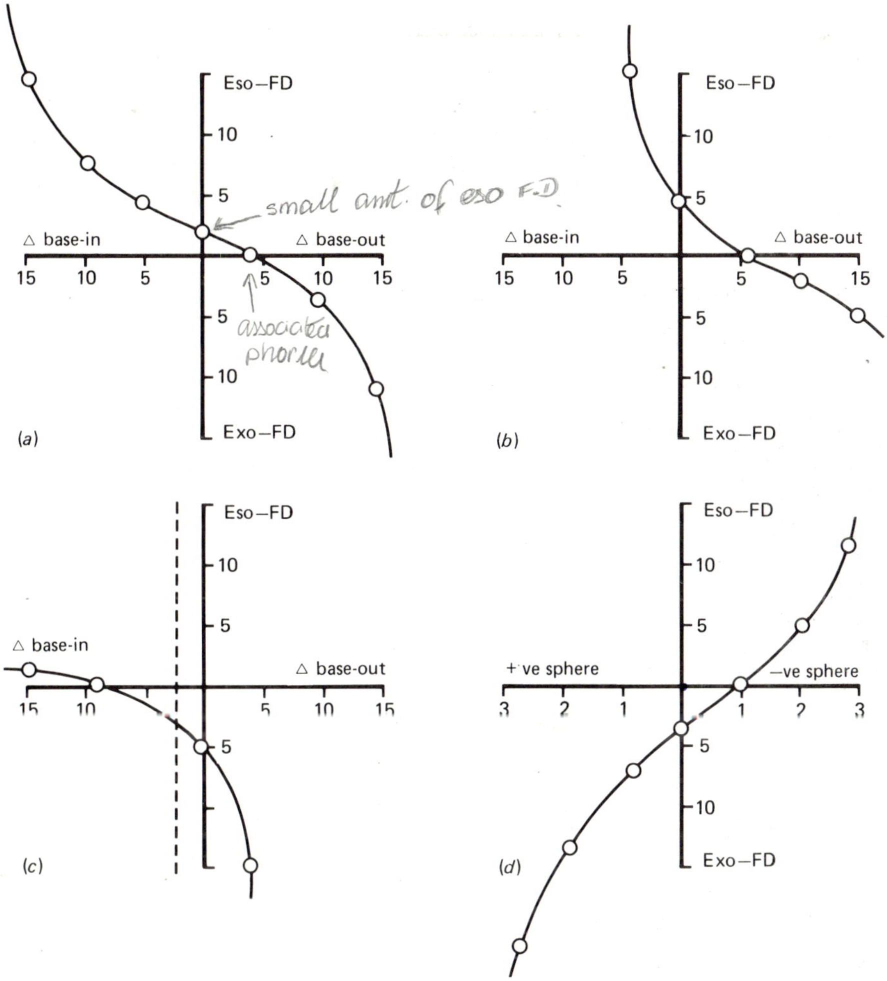

Figure 3.4. Fixation disparity curves: fixation disparity is plotted vertically in minutes of arc and, in the first three curves, the prism power before the eyes in prism dioptres is plotted horizontally. (a) Type I, the most usual curve; (b) Type II, curve in esophoria; (c) Type III, curve in exophoria; (d) fixation disparity plotted against spherical lens power before both eyes (dioptres) for near vision. See also text

range of lower power prisms, but with the higher powers of prism, it rises steeply. Eventually, diplopia would occur at the limit of the prism vergences. Even without the ability to measure the fixation disparity, and therefore plot the curve, this is an interesting clinical concept.

It is suggested that if the patient's normal fixation lies in the flatter part of the curve, it is likely that the heterophoria will be compensated (Sheedy and Saladin, 1978). This is the case in *Figure 3.4(a),* where a small amount of esophoric fixation disparity is present – where the curve cuts the *y*-axis. The associated phoria is also small – where the curve cuts the *x*-axis. In *Figure 3.4(b)*, the curve is placed further towards the right-hand (base-out) side of the figure. This illustrates a case of decompensated esophoria. The fixation disparity and the associated phoria is higher. It will also be appreciated that the base-in prism part of the curve is closer to the y-axis. This means that the base-in prism vergence must be less, and the base-out relatively greater, which is to say that the prism vergences are unbalanced. *Figure 3.4(c)* shows a similar plot, but for exophoria.

If a relieving prism were to be prescribed, it would bring the patient's fixation into the flatter part of the curve. For example, in the case illustrated in *Figure 3.4(c)*, for exophoria, 3^{Δ} base-in vergence would mean that the patient would be operating from the position of the dotted line rather than the actual y-axis. Here, the fixation disparity and associated phoria are less.

Fixation disparity can also be changed by using positive or negative spheres to bring about changes in accommodation. This occurs because of the accommodation–convergence relationship. *Figure 3.4(d)* shows an example of plotting the changes in fixation disparity (y-axis) against the changes in spherical lens power

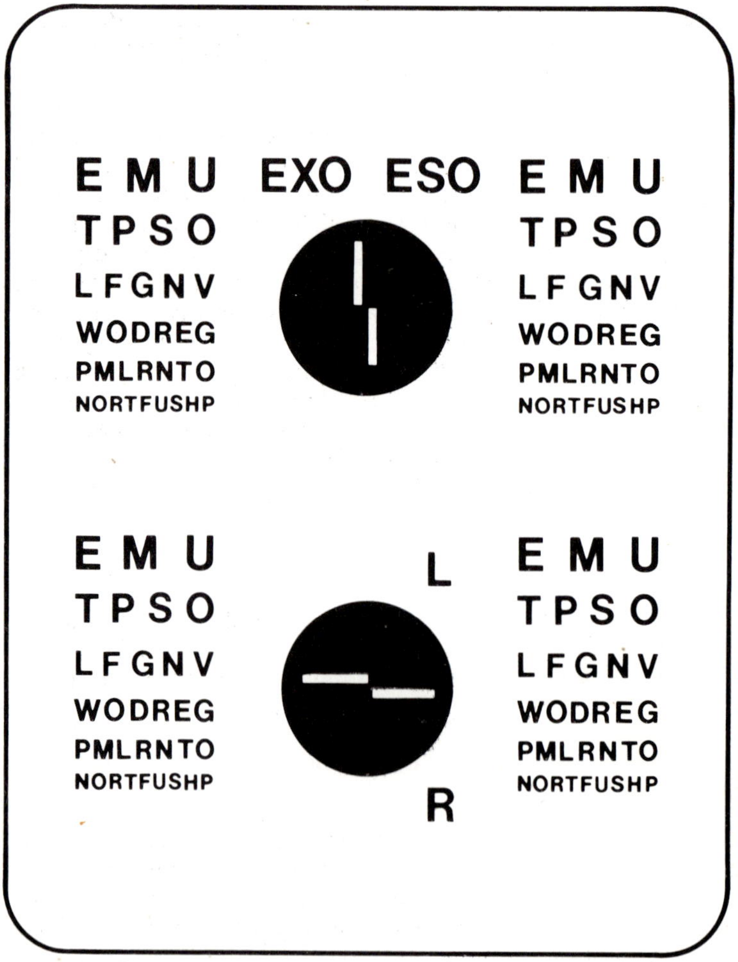

Figure 3.5. The Sheedy disparometer – an example of a disparity test which has no central fixation lock. This apparatus allows the measurement of the actual disparity, i.e. the amount of central misalignment, as well as the associated phoria or degree of prism required to relieve the disparity

(x-axis). In some cases, it is preferable to prescribe spherical lenses rather than prism relief. For example, in the case of a previously uncorrected hyperope, the correction for the hyperopia would be given. In other cases, adjustments to the spherical correction may be given instead of prism relief (see Chapter 4).

The curves shown in *Figure 3.4* were plotted using a device like the disparometer shown in *Figure 3.5*. It should be noted that this differs from the Mallett units in that there is no central or fixation lock. Some authorities doubt that the term 'fixation disparity' can be really applied where there is no binocular fixation point. In this method, the fusion lock is parafoveal (as it is in previously mentioned TIB). The result of using a peripheral lock will be that the degree of fixation disparities obtained will be greater as the Panum's areas are larger in the periphery. In the patient's everyday vision, a central fixation lock is always available. We are concerned in clinical assessment to explore whether the patient's heterophoria is compensated under normal circumstances. It is therefore important that the fusion lock should be within the parafoveal area. The disparometer may be considered to fulfil this. In some cases there will be foveal suppression, and in these patients the lock will be provided by the parafoveal regions, and fixation disparity will be larger; hence the importance of knowing if there is suppression.

All methods of detecting or measuring fixation disparity involve slightly abnormal circumstances which do not coincide with everyday vision. It is therefore important that immediately before investigating disparity the patient should undertake a few moments of binocular vision, such as reading a line of letters binocularly for distance or a few lines of print for near. The Mallett near-vision unit provides printed passages round the near-fixation disparity test for this purpose.

The Zeiss Polatest also provides a range of targets designed to analyse the compensation of the heterophoria. These include acuity and steroscopic tests, and fixation disparity is detected and the associated phoria measured using more peripheral areas, so that the fixation disparity is greater than with tests using parafoveal locks. Both the distance and near Polatests, however, incorporate a very full range of targets, and the designers claim that this allows a greater degree of analysis of binocular vision (Haase, 1962: Pickwell, 1977; 1979).

To summarize on the significance of fixation disparity, the indications that decompensated heterophoria may be present are:

(1) *Fixation disparity* is of a degree greater than normal for the type of apparatus used and it increases under stress.
(2) *Associated phoria* is greater than normal, i.e. a larger than usual prism is required to neutralize the fixation disparity; over 1^{Δ}: or 2^{Δ} for presbyopes.
(3) *Opposing prism vergence* is low and the prism produces a sharp rise in the degree of fixation disparity, quickly leading to diplopia.

Suppression tests

If binocular vision continues under stress for some months, it appears that very small suppression areas occur within the foveal region; that is, during binocular vision little bits of the central field of one eye are inhibited by the mismatch in the slightly misplaced images. The rest of the retina appears to function normally. This suppression does not occur in physiological fixation disparity so it is an added sign of decompensated heterophoria.

Foveal suppression areas can be detected by tests like that on the Mallett Near

Vision Unit, (*Figure 3.3c*), in which some of the letters are crossed polarized to be seen monocularly. If there is suppression, some letters will not be read by the patient.

Stereoscopic tests

The value of stereoscopic tests, or stereotests, in routine examination is two-fold. First, they help to establish that binocular vision is present, and to assess its quality. Where there is central suppression, amblyopia or decompensated heterophoria, the stereoscopic perception may be poor or absent. The second use for stereoscopic tests is to help in assessing a patient's ability to undertake some visual task which requires a good degree of depth perception. However, it must be remembered that clinical methods of testing stereopsis do not necessarily relate to everyday visual tasks. Indeed, they do not relate to each other, as other factors influence performance in these tests (Hall, 1982). Clinical stereoscopic tests, therefore, need to be interpreted with caution in respect to their second function of assessing everyday depth perception.

Where decompensated heterophoria is suspected, the most convenient way of assessing stereopsis in the normal clinical routine is to use one of the stereoscopic tests incorporated in a near-vision test unit (Mallett, 1964). There are, however, many specifically designed stereoscopic tests. A selection of these is shown in *Figure 14.2* on page 144.

Binocular acuity

Normally the binocular acuity will be slightly better than either of the monocular acuities. However, if there is fixation disparity, the lack of a central foveal image in one or both eyes may result in the binocular acuity being the same or worse than the best monocular acuity. This may be detected as the occluder is removed after the monocular refractions (see page 32). The binocular acuity should also be carefully measured. One aspect of the Polatest design is that it provides a lot of

TABLE 3.2. Summary of main factors in assessing compensation of heterophoria

Heterophoria likely to be compensated if:	*Heterophoria likely to decompensated if:*
No symptoms are present due to the heterophoria	Symptoms are present (or foveal suppression is demonstrated)
Quick, smooth recovery after dissociation	Slow or hesitant recovery
Refractive error previously fully corrected	Significant refractive error previously uncorrected
Stable binocular vision to partial dissociation tests	Binocular vision easily breaks down
Balanced prism vergences	Low or unbalanced prism vergences
Exact foveal fixation in binocular vision	Fixation disparity and/or high associated phoria
No foveal suppression	Foveal suppression likely
Good stereopsis	Poor stereopsis
Binocular acuity better than monocular	Binocular acuity poor

lines of higher acuity letters so that the binocular acuity can be compared critically with the monocular (Pickwell, 1977). This can be done with most letter charts.

The evaluation of heterophoria occurs as the routine examination proceeds. It is not usually a process that has to be added on to the routine. The symptoms may indicate quite early that decompensated heterophoria is one of the possible anomalies. The cover test may further suggest this possibility, and the subjective aspect of binocular examination eventually confirms the diagnosis. There is no single test that will provide a conclusive diagnosis in all cases. A summary of the main factors to be considered is given in *Table 3.2*.

References

DAVIS, F. O. (1937). An analysis of some direction investigation. *Dioptric Review*, **39,** 296–312

HAASE, H.-J. (1962). Binocular testing and distance correction with the Berlin Polatest (transl. W. Baldwin). *Journal of the American Optometric Association*, **34,** 115–124

HALL, C. (1982). Relation between clinical stereotests. *Ophthalmic and Physiological Optics*, **2,** 135–143

HUMPHRISS, D. and WOODRUFF, E. W. (1962). Refraction by immediate contrast. *British Journal of Physiological Optics*, **19,** 15–23

MALLETT, R. J. F. (1964). The investigation of heterophoria at near and a new fixation disparity technique. *The Optician*, **148,** 547–551

MALLETT, R. J. F. (1966a). A fixation disparity test for distance use. *The Optician*, **152,** 1–4

MALLETT, R. J. F. (1966b). The investigation of ocular motor imbalances, Part 1. *The Ophthalmic Optician*, **6**(12), 586–596

MALLETT, R. F. J. (1966c). The investigation of occular motor imbalance. Part 2. *The Ophthalmic Optician*, **6**(13), 654–657

MALLETT, R. F. J. (1979). Effect of fixation disparity (letter to Editor). *The Ophthalmic Optician*, **19,** 818–819

MITCHELL, D. W. A. (1953). Investigation of binocular difficulties. *British Journal of Physiological Optics*, **10,** 1

MORGAN, M. W. (1944). The clinical aspects of accommodation and convergence. *American Journal of Optometry*, **21,** 301–313

MORGAN, M. W. (1960). The Turville infinity balance test. *Journal of the American Optometric Association*, **31,** 447–451

OGLE, K. N. (1950). *Researches in Binocular Vision*. W. B. Saunders, Philadelphia and London, pp. 68–93

PERCIVAL, A. S. (1892). The relation of convergence to accommodation and its practical bearing. *Ophthalmologic Review*, **11,** 313–328

PICKWELL, L. D. (1965). Average prism-vergences (unpublished)

PICKWELL, L. D. (1977). Binocular vision: the Berlin outlook. *The Optician*, **174**(8), 11, 35

PICKWELL, L. D. (1979). The effect of fixation disparity. *The Ophthalmic Optician*, **19,** 709, 716

PICKWELL, L. D. and FREIER, BRONWYN (1983). Physiological exophoria. *Ophthalmic and Physiological Optics*, **3**(3), 267–272

PICKWELL, D., JENKINS, T. and YEKTA, A. A. (1987). The effect on fixation disparity and associated heterophoria of reading at an abnormally close distance. *Ophthalmic and Physiological Optics,* **7**(4), 345–347

PICKWELL, L. D. and STOCKLEY, L. A. F. (1960). The position of the retinal image at the limits of fusion. *British Journal of Physiological Optics*, **17**(2), 89–94

PICKWELL, L. D., YEKTA, A. A. and JENKINS, T. C. A. (1987). The effect of reading in low illumination on fixation disparity. *American Journal of Optometry,* **64**(7), 513–518

SCHOR, C. M. (1979). The relation between fusional eye movements and fixation disparity. *Vision Research,* **19**(12), 1359–1367

SHEARD, C. (1930). Zones of ocular comfort. *American Journal of Optometry*, **7,** 9–25

SHEEDY, J. E. and SALADIN, J. J. (1978). Association of symptoms with measurements of oculomotor deficiencies. *American Journal of Optometry*, **55,** 670–676

TURVILLE, A. E. (1946). *Outline of Infinity Balance*. Raphael, London

YEKTA, A. A., JENKINS, T. and PICKWELL, D. (1987). The clinical assessment of binocular vision before and after a working day. *Ophthalmic and Physiological Optics,* **7**(4), 349–352

4

Management of heterophoria: basic principles

Before dealing with the individual heterophoric conditions in the next three chapters, this chapter outlines the basic principles of management.

Following the investigation of binocular vision and the total findings to reach a diagnosis, a decision must be made regarding the best course of action to assist the patient – the management of the case. In general, there are five possible lines of action. One or more of these may help in clearing up the symptoms of the binocular anomaly. Normally, they would be considered in the following order:

(1) Remove the cause of decompensation.
(2) Correct the refractive error.
(3) Give orthoptic treatment.
(4) Prescribe prism relief.
(5) Refer to another practitioner.

Although it is logical to consider them in this order, it may be that some are not appropriate or possible in a particular case. Sometimes only one course of action is going to comprise the primary or sole treatment of the case. For example, in many cases of decompensated heterophoria, the refractive correction by itself will result in the phoria becoming compensated and no further action will be necessary. In other cases, where there is the possibility of active disease or pathology, or of recent injury, referral will be the first priority and other possibilities cannot be pursued until appropriate medical attention has been given.

Removal of cause of decompensation

Consideration must be given to those general factors that put stress on the visual system or on the general well-being of the patient. These factors are discussed in Chapter 1. It will be obvious that all the treatment will aim at removing the cause of the decompensation, and therefore the other four options may also contribute to this. However, there are some factors that contribute to binocular anomalies which do not come under the other headings. For example, a patient working long hours at excessively close work in poor illumination will need to give consideration to proper working conditions, and will be advised accordingly. In some cases, improving the visual working will be all that is required to restore compensation of the heterophoria.

Immediate removal of some of these gene
be possible, as in some instances of poor g
reliance must then be placed on the other o

Correction of refractive error

The importance of the spectacle correction h
high percentage of cases, decompensated heterophoria becomes compensated when a refractive correction is given. It may improve binocular vision for one or more of the following reasons:

(1) *Accommodation–convergence relationship*. This is important in the management of heterophoria. Uncorrected spherical error may result in an abnormal degree of accommodation. This will be excessive in hyperopia and, for near vision, it will be less than normal in myopia. Because of the link of accommodation to convergence, this can result in stress on convergence.

The general rule is that, for esophoria and hyperopia, a full correction be given. A binocular addition of a small sphere may be accepted without blurring distance vision, even if it was not manifest during the monocular refractions. This small addition should be incorporated in the prescription if there is decompensated esophoria. When spectacles are prescribed for near vision only, a further binocular addition is sometimes considered (see Chapter 5).

For esophoria with myopia, a full correction is required to give clear distance vision, but care must be taken not to give an overcorrection; an undercorrection of 0.5 D may be tolerated.

In cases of decompensated exophoria and myopia, a slight overcorrection can be considered if the patient is young enough for no stress to be put on the amplitude of accommodation. For exophoric patients with hyperopia, care must be taken that the correction does not contribute to the phoria becoming decompensated; a partial correction can be considered if this is likely.

(2) *Blurring*. If it occurs in one or both eyes, blurring will make binocular vision more difficult. This is particularly important in high astigmatism, and care must be taken to ensure an accurate astigmatic correction.

(3) *Anisometropia*. When anisometropia requires different amounts of accommodation it produces differences in blurring, it can also be important in making the heterophoria decompensated. In some cases, the differences in the refractive error between the two eyes is gross and needs particular attention. Chapter 9 is devoted to dealing with the particular difficulties that can arise in these cases.

In other cases, care must be taken to ensure that the refractive correction is properly balanced, either by a retinoscopic method or subjectively. The methods are described briefly in Chapter 3.

Orthoptic treatment

Usually, the effect of the refractive correction on the heterophoria is assessed before orthoptic exercises are considered. The patient is asked to wear the glasses for about 1 month to see if this will alleviate the symptoms. In those cases where there is no refractive error, orthoptics may be considered immediately.

In general, decompensated heterophoria responds well to orthoptic treatment. Some conditions and some patients seem to be more amenable to orthoptics. Particular types of heterophoria are discussed in the next five chapters, which indicate the conditions likely to respond to exercises. As far as the patients are concerned, younger ones are more likely to have a successful outcome. In decompensated heterophoria, patients between the ages of 12 and 35 years respond better, but sometimes orthoptics can be successful outside this range. Patients under 12 years are seen less frequently with decompensated heterophoria. In some conditions, presbyopic patients sometimes benefit from simple orthoptic exercises.

Another factor affecting the success of orthoptic treatment is the incentive of the patient. Sometimes the patient is not prepared to give the time and effort necessary. Where the symptoms are marked, the incentive will be high. In conditions where suppression has intervened to lessen the symptoms, the disturbance to binocular vision may be marked, but there may be less incentive for the patient to carry out the exercises. Teenage patients may have a deal of school work and a broad range of other interests competing for their time. Some patients will readily undertake the exercises and will conscientiously carry them out to the end. Others will start enthusiastically, but prove to have insufficient patience to complete the course. Binocular anomalies will not respond to orthoptic exercises that are insufficiently carried out. The practitioner's enthusiasm, however, may prove infectious and often makes all the difference between success and failure.

It is important to understand the nature of orthoptic exercises. Orthoptics is a learning process, in the same way as motor skills are learned. There are many motor skills which we may require during life. They vary from such things as learning to ride a bicycle to touch-typing. They require practice until the motor and sensory systems are co-ordinated to undertake them automatically. At first, a good deal of thought and concentration is required, but in time they become 'conditioned reflexes'. Orthoptics consists of re-educating the visual reflexes and acquiring proper visual habits. Orthoptic exercises are not concerned with strengthening the power of the individual eye muscles, but re-establishing correct muscles and sensory co-ordination.

The patient must have sufficient intelligence to understand what is required, and the exercises be explained simply enough to be understood. The patient does not need to understand the exact nature of the binocular anomaly, but only what he or she is required to do. However, with older patients it may help in maintaining interest and co-operation if the broad aims of the particular treatment can be explained.

The exact type of orthoptic treatment that may be given may vary with the particular type of heterophoria present, and this is discussed with the various types of heterophoria in the following chapters.

Prism relief

Where orthoptic treatment is inappropriate because of age or ill-health, or due to lack of time or incentive on the part of the patient, prism relief may be considered. As mentioned above, some heterophoric conditions are unlikely to respond to orthoptics, and relieving prisms are more appropriate. Hyperphoria is of this type. Therefore, in decompensated hyperphoria prism relief is more usual.

Relieving prisms are more applicable to exophoria than to esophoria. In decompensated esophoria, small positive additions to the spherical part of the prescription will often make the phoria compensated, and base-out prisms are seldom needed.

The power of the prism to be prescribed is the minimum which just allows the heterophoria to become compensated. This is always less than the degree of the phoria measured by a dissociation method. It is more likely to be the degree of the associated phoria. Indeed, the Mallett units are designed to give the correct degree of dissociation, so that the weakest prism which neutralizes the fixation disparity is the appropriate prism to incorporate in the prescription (Mallett, 1966). The prism power can also be assessed by finding the weakest prism which produces a quick and smooth recovery movement to the cover test. Indeed, any of the clinical tests described in Chapter 3 for assessing compensation may help in prescribing prisms.

Adaptation to prisms occurs with most patients. When the prism is first placed before the eyes, it will relieve the heterophoria by the magnitude of the prism, and also lessen the fixation disparity. After several minutes, the binocular system adapts to the prism, and the heterophoria and the fixation disparity return to the original value (Carter, 1963; 1965). It appears, however, that patients with abnormal binocular vision which causes symptoms do not adapt, or only partially adapt, to prisms (North and Henson, 1981). Eventually, a method could be developed which uses this poor adaptation to prism as a clinical method to help the detection of decompensated heterophoria and gives further indications on when to prescribe prisms. It has also been shown that some patients who had abnormal adaptation to prisms before receiving orthoptic treatment have normal prism adaptation after treatment (North and Henson, 1982).

Referral

It is obvious that, under some circumstances, a patient must be referred or a report sent to another practitioner. It is important to be guided in this decision, not only by the law or local regulations which may require referral, but by what is in the best interests of each patient. Patients should be referred if:

(a) there is a factor contributing to the decompensation of the heterophoria which requires attention by another practitioner, and which cannot be given by the optometrist – for example, the patient's health may have deteriorated, causing the decompensation;
(b) the cause of the decompensation is suspected to be pathological or a recent head injury;
(c) the heterophoria is unlikely to respond to any of the approaches described in this chapter, but the symptoms persist.

All practitioners need to appreciate the limitations to their own field of expertise, experience and competence, and to refer patients in their own interest as well as that of the patient.

In summary, the management of heterophoria consists of identifying the factors contributing to the decompensation and removing as many of these as possible. In many cases the correction of the refractive error will achieve this end. Sometimes it is necessary to improve binocular functions by orthoptics or to give prism relief. If the patient is suffering some more general stress or poor health, referral to an appropriate practitioner may be required.

In general symptoms due to heterophoria can be said to be the result in some change in the patient's circumstances which has contributed to stress on the binocular vision; for example, additional close work, or poor health. This change is likely to be fairly recent: long standing problems either have developed suppression of one eye to alleviate the symptoms or the patient will be well aware of the problem over a long time. However the change is recent in most cases and it is therefore likely that it can be identified. Most decompensated heterophoria has become decompensated due to stress on the visual system or on the general well-being of the patient as described in Chapter 1 on page 7. This means not only can it be identified but that also it may be removed or relieved by one of the five lines of action outlined above.

References

CARTER, D. B. (1963). Effect of prolonged wearing of prisms. *American Journal of Optometry*, **40**(5), 265–273

CARTER, D. B. (1965). Fixation disparity and heterophoria following prolonged wearing of prisms. *American Journal of Optometry*, **42**(3), 141–153

MALLETT, R. F. (1966). The investigation of ocular motor imbalance. *The Ophthalmic Optician*, Part 1, **6**, 586–596; Part 2, **6**, 654–657

NORTH, R. V. and HENSON, D. B. (1981). Adaptation to prism induced heterophoria in subjects with abnormal binocular vision or asthenopia. *American Journal of Optometry*, **58**(9), 746–752

NORTH, R. V. and HENSON, D. B. (1982). Effect of orthoptics upon the ability of patients to adapt to prism induced heterophoria. *American Journal of Optometry*, **59**, 983–990

LTC

5

Esophoric conditions

Most esophoria is 'accommodative', in that a major part of its aetiology (or cause) is excessive accommodation resulting from uncorrected hyperopia or from excessive close work. As a result of the accommodation/convergence linkage, the excessive accommodation produces excessive convergence. Some eso-deviations do not have this accommodative factor and are then known as 'non-accommodative' or sometimes as anatomical esophoria or esotropia.

Esophoria can be classified according to whether the convergence is greater for distance of for near vision, or if it is the same for both:

(1) *Divergence weakness type* – shows decompensated esophoria for distance vision. In near vision, the heterophoria will be compensated. In older patients, there will be the expected degree of physiological exophoria, reducing the measured degree of esophoria for near vision.
(2) *Convergence excess* – characterized by an increase in the degree of esophoria for near vision. There is usually a small degree of compensated heterophoria for distance vision, and a higher degree of esophoria which is decompensated for near vision. This is in contrast to the normal physiological exophoria.
(3) *Basic (or mixed) type* – shows decompensated esophoria of about the same degree in distance and in near vision. The methods of investigation and management that apply to both divergence weakness esophoria and to convergence excess esophoria will apply to basic esophoria. A separate section on basic esophoria is therefore not included.

Divergence weakness esophoria

Aetiology

UNCORRECTED HYPEROPIA

This is the most common cause for decompensated esophoria in distance vision – accommodative esophoria. It is usually decreased by the spectacle correction to the extent that it becomes compensated.

MUSCLE TONUS

When in the adductors (medial recti muscles), muscle tonus is often a factor, particularly in children and teenage patients.

ANATOMICAL FACTORS

Those such as abnormal orbital shape, lengths of check ligaments, muscles insertions, etc., are thought to contribute to esophoria in some patients. There is no evidence to show that these change in adult life, except for injury. If esophoria becomes decompensated, therefore, it is because other factors have intervened: poor health, deteriorated working conditions, etc. The anatomical factors may, however, explain why some patients' esophoria decompensates, whereas in others it does not in similar circumstances.

EXCITABLE OR 'NEUROTIC' TEMPERAMENTS

The esophoria in these cases may be variable with the emotional state and level of anxiety, being compensated one day and decompensated the next. It is also aggravated by stimulants.

ANOXAEMIA

Lack of oxygen (anoxaemia) in patients who work in stuffy atmospheres for long periods may cause divergence weakness esophoria to become decompensated.

PATHOLOGY

Pathological disturbances, particularly those affecting the central nervous system, will usually cause incomitant esophoria which will tend to break down into squint in one direction of gaze. Incomitancy is not the subject of this chapter, but is dealt with in Chapter 16.

Investigation

A routine examination of the eye and vision is carried out in each case. In this type of esophoria, particular attention can be given to the undermentioned factors:

(1) *Symptoms*, which are usually associated with distance vision unless there is high hyperopia, which will accentuate the symptoms for close work. The symptoms will be associated with prolonged use of the eyes, and will be less or absent in the morning unless there is a pathological cause. The symptoms are likely to be headaches in the frontal area, sometimes intermittent diplopia and blurred near vision if uncorrected hyperopia is present.
(2) *Refraction*, which is very important in divergence weakness type esophoria because of the association with uncorrected hyperopia.
(3) *Decompensation tests*, which will be the most important aspect in the investigation. The skills required to assess compensation are fully described in Chapter 3. Measurement of the heterophoria by the cover test or subjective dissociation tests will show a higher degree for distance than for near vision.

Management

REMOVAL OF CAUSE OF DECOMPENSATION

The factors likely to put stress on the visual system or on the general well-being of the patient should be considered. These are described in Chapter 1. Consider particularly the patient's visual working conditions and the possibility of poor ventilation being a contributory cause in this type of esophoria.

REFRACTIVE CORRECTION

Uncorrected hyperopia is the most common cause of decompensation in this type of esophoria, and therefore the spectacle correction is most likely to remove the symptoms. In many cases, no other form of treatment is required. A full correction for the hyperopia is given. In children and young adults, a cycloplegic refraction may be considered if variable refractive findings make it difficult to assess the refractive error or if latent hyperopia is suspected.

The patients should be asked to wear the correction constantly for distance and near vision for about a month, and then tests for compensation repeated if symptoms persist. Where the spectacles clear up the symptoms and the esophoria becomes compensated, the spectacle correction should be worn when the patient finds the need. This will depend on the degree of the hyperopia and the stress on binocular vision created by the visual conditions.

In some cases the esophoria is not changed by a hyperopic correction or there is found to be no refractive error – the esophoria is non-accommodative. Consideration should then be given to orthoptic treatment or relieving prisms. Occasionally, myopes have decompensated esophoria for distance vision. The lowest correction is given that is consistent with good distance acuity.

ORTHOPTIC TREATMENT

If the decompensation of divergence weakness type esophoria persists after consideration has been given to the general decompensating factors and the spectacle correction, orthoptic exercises may be considered.

Teaching an appreciation of physiological diplopia has been found to be useful in this condition. The patient is asked to look at a small isolated object (not confused with background details) at a distance of 3–6 m. A second object, such as a pencil, is held on the median line at about 40 cm from the eyes. The patient is encouraged to notice that this second object is seen in physiological diplopia as long as fixation is maintained on the distance one. When this has been appreciated, fixation is changed to the near object, and physiological diplopia of the distance one is observed. The patient is then encouraged to alternate between fixing the distance object with crossed physiological diplopia of the near one, and fixing the near object with uncrossed physiological diplopia of the distant one. A pause of several seconds must be made with each change of fixation, or confusion results. This exercise in vergence co-ordination seems to be particularly useful in young patients.

Exercises to increase the divergent amplitude of prism vergences (the negative fusional reserve) and/or the positive relative accommodation are also of help in this type of esophoria, and often the main orthoptic therapy. A range of suitable exercises is described in Chapter 8.

RELIEVING PRISMS

Prism relief in esophoria is required only for a minority of cases. The symptoms in most cases are relieved by the spectacle correction or by orthoptic treatment. Prisms may be considered when orthoptic treatment has been tried and found not to be successful, or where it is inappropriate because of the patient's age, poor health, unwillingness or inability to give the time required. The power of the prism required is that which is likely to make the esophoria compensated, as assessed by the method described in Chapter 4. In general, it will be the lowest prism power which will give no disparity on the fixation disparity test, or a smooth prompt recovery on the cover test.

REFERRAL

This will be the first consideration when a pathological cause is suspected, but it is unlikely that surgery will help in other cases.

Convergence excess esophoria

As the name suggests, this type of esophoria is low in degree for distance vision, but on converging for near vision the convergence impulses seem to be unusually high. This results in a high degree of esophoria for near vision.

Aetiology

EXCESSIVE ACCOMMODATIVE EFFORT

This is usually the main factor, and may be caused by uncorrected hyperopia, latent hyperopia, spasm of accommodation or by pseudomyopia. Another frequent cause is very prolonged work at an excessively close working distance.

HIGH AC/A RATIO

The accommodative convergence/accommodation, or AC/A, ratio is often a factor in producing convergence excess esophoria. The ratio is a measure of the effect of a change in accommodation on the convergence. It is expressed as the change in convergence (in prism dioptres) for each dioptre change in accommodation. This is normally about 4^{Δ}/1 D (just expressed as an AC/A ratio of 4). When it is high (over 6), accommodation for near vision will result in the excess of convergence. Convergence excess rarely occurs with a low AC/A ratio.

HYSTERICAL REACTION

Convergence excess can also be present as a hysterical reaction. When this occurs it is usually in young energetic patients, and it is typically accompanied by some psychological stress or anxiety; for example, school examination pressures or relationship difficulties.

INCIPIENT PRESBYOPIA

This can occasionally result in convergence excess, due to the high ciliary muscle effort needed to produce adequate accommodation.

Investigation

Each case of convergence excess esophoria will require a full routine examination and probably a cycloplegic refraction. Particular attention should be given to the undermentioned factors:

(1) *Symptoms* which are usually associated with prolonged use of the eyes in near vision. Sometimes they are so severe as to render close work impossible for more than short periods. Frontal headache, ocular fatigue and blurred near vision are usual symptoms. Sometimes difficulty is experienced in refocusing the eyes for distance vision after a lot of close work.

(2) *Refraction*, which may show variable and unreliable results. It may be seen during the retinoscopy; neutralization appearing at one moment and 'with' or 'against' movement the next, without any test-lens change. This is a sign of active accommodation, and may indicate the presence of latent hyperopia. Another sign of latent error is a lower subjective result that than shown in retinoscopy. These are clear indications that a cycloplegic refraction is required to reveal any latent error or spasm of accommodation that may accompany convergence excess esophoria. Occasionally, the spasm is such that pseudomyopia occurs. This is usually of low degree, but can be as high as 10 D. Where myopia occurs in a young patient with high esophoria for near vision, the possibility of spasm should be explored by cycloplegic examination.

(3) *A gradient test*, which may be considered as giving useful information in convergence excess. It is one of a number of ways of measuring the AC/A ratio, and is the usual method in this condition. The degree of esophoria for near vision is measured in the normal way and with the spectacle correction in place. It is then measured with binocular positive additions to change the accommodation. The change in convergence per dioptre of accommodation is then found. For example, if the heterophoria measurement with the prescription is 6^{Δ} esophoria, with an addition of +1.00 DS is 1^{Δ}, and with +2.00 DS is 4^{Δ} exophoria, the vergence is changing by 5^{Δ} per dioptre of accommodation, that is, an AC/A ratio of 5.

(4) *A cover test and fixation disparity test* for near vision, which will indicate decompensation of the heterophoria at near.

Management

REMOVAL OF CAUSE OF DECOMPENSATION

It is usually necessary to restrict the patient's close work and/or to increase the working distance. In many cases of convergence excess, the working distance has become unnecessarily close, due to bad visual habits. Patients acquire the habit of working excessively close during childhood, when the amplitude of accommodation was sufficient to permit this without symptoms, but on reaching the age when the amplitude is reduced, stress occurs and becomes the cause of the convergence excess (see above). Most patients with this condition are, as might be expected, between 14 and 20 years of age. The onset will vary with the amount of close work and the working distance, as well as with the degree of uncorrected refractive error. It may also be brought on by a marked increase in the amount of close work; for example, due to an approaching school examination period, or leaving school for a clerical job with longer hours of sustained near vision.

In some cases, changing the visual habits to require the patient to employ a more appropriate working distance will clear up the symptoms with no other treatment. A distance of 35–40 cm should be regarded as a minimum. It is not always easy for patients to acquire new visual habits when the concentration is on the job in hand. It is usually necessary for them to ask someone else to keep reminding them of the required working distance.

REFRACTIVE CORRECTION

The full hyperopic correction found by the cycloplegic refraction is prescribed, to be worn for distance and near vision in the first place (allowance is made for tonus if appropriate). With this correction, the patient's distance vision may be blurred at first, but it should clear as the latent error becomes manifest. This may occur quite quickly, after half an hour, say, or it may require several days.

In any case, the patient should be seen again after wearing the correction for 2 weeks, and the symptoms and decompensation reassessed. If the symptoms have cleared, the glasses should continue to be worn for reading and other close work, and for distance vision, as required to maintain relief of the symptoms. In cases of high hyperopia, this may involve continued constant wear.

Bifocals, with a reading addition that relieves the decompensation of the esophoria for near vision, are sometimes prescribed. The addition can be found with the gradient test method, or by adding positive spheres until the cover test or fixation disparity indicate compensation. However, this approach to convergence excess is seldom necessary in patients over the age of 14 years, and for younger patients it is better restricted to those cases where orthoptic treatment is not possible or not successful in relieving the symptoms.

Sometimes convergence excess breaks down into a squint for near vision. In these cases, bifocals may be appropriate if binocular vision is restored when the patient looks through the segment. In any case, the bifocal addition is gradually reduced as the condition becomes more stable, and bifocals are not considered as a long-term correction. Patients with bifocals should be checked every 3–6 months, with a view to reducing the addition. Bifocals are not suitable as a method of management if the AC/A ratio is low.

Where convergence excess occurs in incipient presbyopia, reading glasses are prescribed.

ORTHOPTIC TREATMENT

If the symptoms persist after the constant wear of the spectacle correction for several weeks, orthoptic exercises may be considered. Exercises that develop the positive relative accommodation are particularly useful. The aim of such exercises is to encourage accommodation without convergence; pairs of negative spheres increasing in power can be placed before the eyes whilst the patient maintains clear single vision. Alternatively, the divergent amplitude of the prism vergence can be developed. In this case the accommodation is unchanged while the eyes diverge. This can be done by a prism vergence exercise. Both exercises can be carried out with a Holmes stereoscope. Details of these exercises are given in the general chapter on exercises (Chapter 8). In the case of convergence excess, the exercises will be carried out for near vision.

RELIEVING PRISMS

This is not appropriate to convergence excess, unless the AC/A ratio is very low – 2 or 3 – which is unusual.

REFERRAL

Medical attention should be sought if pathology is suspected, or appropriate help can be sought where there is psychological stress.

6

Exophoric conditions

Although it has been shown that divergence is actively stimulated (Breinin, 1957), exophoria appears to be a much more passive condition than esophoria. This may be because the position of anatomical rest is relatively divergent, because divergence has been thought to be a relaxation of convergence associated with a relaxation of accommodation, and because the eyes do not diverge beyond the parallel in normal vision. High tonic impulses to the abductors do not seem to be considered such a major factor in most exophoria in the way that high muscle tonus of the adductors contribute to esophoria. For near vision, factors that produce excessive convergence in children can even mask a basic exophoric deviation.

Exophoria can be considered under four headings:

(1) *Convergence weakness exophoria* – shows decompensated exophoria for near vision, but not for distance. For distance, there is usually a smaller degree of exophoria which is compensated. This type will be dealt with together with basic exophoria.
(2) *Divergence excess* – in its typical form this is an intermittent divergent squint for distance vision with compensated exophoria for near vision. Sometimes it is defined as an exo-deviation of 15^{Δ} greater for distance vision than for near.
(3) *Basic (or mixed) exophoria* – is the type of exophoria in which the degree does not differ significantly with the fixation distance.
(4) *Convergence insufficiency* – is an inability to sustain sufficient convergence for comfortable near vision. Although this may be considered to be an anomaly of convergence rather than heterophoria in the strictest sense, it will be considered in this chapter with the exophoric conditions.

Basic and convergence weakness exophoria

Although basic exophoria and exophoria for near vision only (convergence weakness type exophoria) may be considered as two different conditions, the methods of examination and management have so much in common that they will be dealt with together. In the investigation and the management of convergence weakness exophoria, thought will need to be given particularly to near vision.

Aetiology

ANATOMICAL FACTORS

These seem to play a large part in most cases of exophoria, possibly because of the normal divergent position of anatomical rest.

HYPERTONICITY OF THE ABDUCTORS

This may be a contributory factor.

MYOPIA

When uncorrected, myopia may build up a false accommodation–convergence relationship for near vision.

AGE

The average phoria for near vision increases with age from the early twenties, becoming about 6^{Δ} exophoria by the age of about 60 years. This is a steady progression which does not increase sharply at the age when presbyopic additions are first prescribed. In most normal people, the degree of exophoria for near vision is increased when the addition is first placed before the eyes, but in a few minutes it decreases to return to the value before the reading addition was used. With normal patients, the physiological exophoria for near vision does not seem to be caused by the reading addition (Freier and Pickwell, 1983). Elderly patients often have decompensated exophoria for near vision.

ABSOLUTE HYPEROPIA

This may be a factor in the cause of exophoria. Patients whose hyperopia is high in comparison with their amplitude of accommodation reach an age when they are no longer able to compensate for their refractive error by accommodating. They allow their accommodation and their convergence to flag, resulting in decompensated exophoria. This can happen in high hyperopia in children, and commonly in low degrees of hyperopia in incipient presbyopes, particularly in people who do not have to undertake a lot of near visual tasks.

SUPPRESSION

Suppression of one eye, which has been acquired because of long periods of using monocular vision, is also a factor. This used to occur in some occupations in which instruments with monocular eyepieces were used. Nowadays, instruments with binocular eyepieces are more often used, so that few patients suffer from an acquired form of suppression.

Investigation

A routine eye examination should be carried out in each case, as described in Chapter 2. Two points should be noted, particularly in this type of exophoria:

(1) *Symptoms*, which are not usually as marked in exophoria as in esophoria. Suppression is more likely to be associated with exophoria and this will lessen the symptoms to some extent. The symptoms are likely to include frontal headache associated with prolonged use of the eyes, ocular fatigue and sometimes intermittent diplopia, particularly for near vision. In old age there is often a high degree of exophoria for near vision which is not accompanied by symptoms.
(2) *A cover test*, which may reveal the exophoria early in the routine examination; particular attention must then be paid to assessment of the compensation, as described in Chapter 3.

Management

REMOVAL OF CAUSE OF DECOMPENSATION

Attention should be given to the patient's working conditions, adequate illumination and the possibility of a visual task involving monocular vision and causing suppression. The patient's general health should also be considered.

REFRACTIVE CORRECTION

In myopia or in absolute hyperopia, the spectacle correction can assist in making the exophoria compensated, and this applies to distance and to near vision anomalies. In hyperopic cases, care needs to be exercised in prescribing, as sometimes the correction increases the symptoms and difficulties. The exophoria should be assessed for compensation with the full correction in place. Sometimes it can be demonstrated quickly that the degree of the exophoria is increased by the correction, and that the binocular vision has become less stable. It should be noted, however, that the exophoria can adapt to the lenses if they are left in place for a few minutes (see above). The assessment needs to be made, therefore, when the lenses have been worn for several minutes. In those cases where the hyperopic correction results in the exophoria becoming decompensated, or if it is likely to so do, a partial correction is given. In the case of a patient who has had no previous glasses, the correction should be reduced by about one-third of the mean spherical error, and the assessment of the exophoria repeated. The correction required is the highest correction that will maintain a compensated exophoria and which will at the same time relieve the symptoms of the hyperopia. In a few cases, this may not be possible, and for these, prism relief or orthoptic treatment can be considered.

In presbyopia, the reading addition should be kept as low as is compatible with adequate near vision, particularly in decompensated exophoria for near vision only – convergence weakness type.

ORTHOPTIC TREATMENT

In patients under the age of about 20 years, orthoptic treatment may be appropriate, depending on the incentive of the patient, the time available, etc. (see Chapter 4 for the general considerations). It may be successful with younger adults if the exophoria has been compensated but due to stress has become decompensated. In such cases, a short course of orthoptic exercises aids the restoration of compensation when the factors of stress have been dealt with.

Where treatment is given, the general plan of this should be:

(1) Treat any suppression that has been demonstrated.

(2) Develop the base-out prism vergences and/or the negative relative accommodation.
(3) Develop a correct appreciation of physiological diplopia.

Examples of exercises appropriate to these objectives are described in Chapter 8.

RELIEVING PRISMS

Prism relief in exophoria cases often proves a simple and effective method of management. It is frequently more appropriate than orthoptic treatment in adult patients.

The power of the prism to incorporate in the prescription is the lowest which will ensure compensation of the exophoria. This can be estimated by repeating the cover test with prism relief in place before the eyes, or by measuring the associated phoria with a Mallett fixation disparity unit. The smallest prism which restores the monocular markers to their central position is prescribed.

There is often a subjective improvement reported by the patient when reading the near-test types with the prism in place, and it may be noticeably worse if the prism is removed.

If there is a small degree of commitant hyperphoria in addition to the exophoria, the relief by vertical prism will help the compensation of the exophoria (London and Wick, 1987).

REFERRAL

Where other methods of relief fail, surgical relief is sometimes considered, but the degree of the exophoria has to be large enough to exceed the accuracy expected.

Divergence excess

Divergence excess shows a large degree of exophoria for distance vision, which in many cases will be found to break down into a divergent squint. For near vision, the heterophoria is less by at least 7^{Δ} (Duane, 1897), and is compensated. The majority of patients with divergence excess are female, and the condition seems to present itself in the mid-teens (Pickwell, 1979). A distinction has been made between 'true divergence excess' and 'simulated divergence excess' (Burian and von Noorden, 1974). In the latter case, it may be considered to be a basic exo-deviation in a young patient with high tonic, accommodative or proximal convergence which obscures the real nature of the deviation for near vision. The high convergence lessens as the patient reaches adult age, and simulated divergence excess then reveals itself to be a basic exo-deviation. This may be important where surgery is to be considered, but non-surgical management may be the same for true and simulated divergence excess in the initial stages. In simulated divergence excess, the management may have to be modified as the patient gets older.

Aetiology

The causes of divergence excess are uncertain, and there has been a good deal of speculation as to the relative importance of the tonic and anatomical factors.

Investigation

The investigation of divergence excess should follow the routine eye examination, giving particular attention to the following points:

(1) *Symptoms*, although patients with divergence excess do not usually complain of any marked subjective symptoms. If asked, they may report that intermittent diplopia has been present for as long as they can remember, but often there is established suppression and this is not reported. Some patients learn to control the deviation for distance by accommodating, and will report some blurred vision as a result. The most usual reason given for presenting for eye examination is that their friends and relatives have noticed the divergence of one eye. This deviation becomes apparent with inattention, and may increase with emotional stress. Bright sunlight is also reported to produce the deviation (Eustace, Weston and Druby, 1973). Patients may therefore report that the deviation is often noticed or that they close one eye in bright light. Poor health or small amounts of alcohol can also produce the deviation.

(2) *A cover test,* which may show decompensated exophoria for distance vision, but sometimes this can appear compensated if the patient is exercising a high level of concentration. If the cover test is repeated, or the alternating cover test carried out, the distance vision deviation increases and the exophoria may break down into a divergent squint. The Maddox rod and compensation tests may also show similar variation for distance vision.

   The V syndrome often accompanies divergence excess (see Chapter 16).

(3) *Refractive error*, which in divergence excess is usually either low hyperopia or myopia (Pickwell, 1979).

(4) *Prism vergences*, which are usually very abnormal in that the base-in amplitude is very high: instead of the average value of 6–9$^{\Delta}$, they may exceed 20$^{\Delta}$. The very divergent position produced by measuring the base-in prism vergence for distance vision is usually accompanied by suppression. This means that in some cases, when the limit of the divergent amplitude is reached, no diplopia is reported and this may give the appearance of a very much higher amplitude, unless the practitioner watches the patient's eyes behind the prism to note the point at which the divergence of one eye ceases.

   The very high base-in prism vergence for distance vision is therefore a major diagnostic feature.

Management

REMOVAL OF CAUSE OF DECOMPENSATION

This is not possible in divergence excess.

REFRACTIVE CORRECTION

Correction of the myopia assists by clearing the blurred distance vision. Where there is a low degree of hyperopia, a correction does not seem to assist, unless it is required to equalize the acuities. Sunglasses or tinted prescription lenses sometimes assist compensation.

ORTHOPTIC TREATMENT

With teenage patients, orthoptic treatment can be very helpful for many with divergence excess. The incentive of the patient may not be very high, as there are often no marked symptoms, but where there is a reasonable level of co-operation, it may be the most appropriate form of management.

Where orthoptic treatment is given, the same three aims given above for basic exophoria are equally appropriate to divergence excess: treat the suppression; develop the base-out prism vergence and/or negative relative accommodation; develop a correct appreciation of physiological diplopia. These aims may be achieved by some of the exercises described in Chapter 8. They may be taken in the above order, or an exercise used which incorporates more than one aim. For example, physiological diplopia can be used in such a way that it develops convergence and relative accommodation, and at the same time it will, by its nature, help in checking suppression. This type of exercise has been found particularly useful in divergence excess.

RELIEVING PRISMS

These are seldom satisfactory in divergence excess, as they disturb near vision.

REFERRAL

Surgery may be considered in cases of simulated divergence excess as the patient gets older and an exo-deviation occurs at all distances of fixation.

Convergence insufficiency

Convergence is essential to binocular vision at near, and therefore any inadequacy is of great clinical importance. Convergence insufficiency has been recognized as a fairly common condition since it was described by von Graefe (1862). It may be defined as an inability to obtain or to maintain sufficient convergence for comfortable binocular vision at near.

Aetiology

DISUSE OF ACCOMMODATIVE CONVERGENCE

This can be a cause of convergence insufficiency. Uncorrected myopes, presbyopes wearing their reading glasses and absolute hyperopes may all make reduced accommodative effort, which results in insufficient convergence because of the accommodation/convergence relationship.

ANATOMICAL FACTORS

Factors such as a large pupillary distance or a divergent position of anatomical rest may contribute.

DEVELOPMENTAL (OR PHYLOGENETIC) FACTORS

These may also play a part: convergence is the most recently developed aspect of binocular vision and may most readily break down under stress.

SQUINT

This can be a contributory cause. It has long been recognized that divergent squint in early life can be a factor (Duane, 1897), but more recently a survey showed that in squinting patients, convergence insufficiency was present in both convergent and divergent deviations in about the same proportions as the general incidence of convergent to divergent squint overall (Pickwell and Hampshire, 1981b).

DISUSE OF AN EYE

Disuse of one eye for any length of time, amblyopia in one eye or a blurred image in one eye can also induce convergence insufficiency, and may be a factor in squint.

VERTICAL HETEROPHORIA

This may cause convergence insufficiency. The hyperphoria may be comitant in some cases, or it may be found to be incomitant and break down into a squint in some direction of gaze or under adverse visual conditions. In the latter case, surgery is suggested before treatment of the convergence inadequacy (Lyle and Wybar, 1967).

GENERAL DEBILITY

Poor general health has been shown to be a factor (Pickwell and Hampshire, 1984). Independent of health, there is a greater incidence with age (Pickwell, 1985), and in urban populations compared to rural (Pickwell, Viggars and Jenkins, 1986).

Metabolic disorders, toxic conditions and local infections or endocrine disorders are important factors. For example, convergence weakness can accompany thyrotoxicosis as an early sign (Moebius's sign).

PARALYSIS OF CONVERGENCE

This can also rarely occur in conditions affecting the brain-stem, in disseminated sclerosis, tabes and in some traumatic conditions. In these cases, there is a sudden onset of diplopia for near vision, and usually other signs and symptoms of the primary condition.

Investigation

In the investigation of convergence insufficiency, particular attention should be paid to the following points:

(1) *Symptoms*, which are usually associated with near vision and consist of tired eyes, intermittent blurring and double vision, and headache. Sometimes patients will report that the symptoms are relieved if one eye is closed or covered. The symptoms are worse if the patient is suffering from tiredness, ill-health, overwork, anxiety, etc., as they are with heterophoria.
(2) *Convergence tests*, which are a major factor in the diagnosis. Two clinical tests are of particular value, and are simple and brief enough to include in a standard routine examination. The methods of application of these tests are described in Chapter 2.

Near point of convergence, which is normally taken as being less than 10 cm from the eyes. It should be observed by the practitioner as the distance at which one eye ceases to converge, and also the point at which the patient reports a doubling of the target as it approaches the eyes. In some cases, no doubling is reported, but the limit of convergence can be seen objectively. This will indicate suppression, which may be the first sign of possible difficulty. Patients whose near point of convergence is between 10 cm and 20 cm may have convergence difficulties. Such patients need to be assessed when any anomaly of jump convergence is known, and normal near visual working distance has been taken into account.

Jump convergence, which is the other aspect for routine investigation. The patient is asked to look at a distance object, and then to change fixation to one held at about 15 cm from the eyes and on the median line. The eyes are observed to see if the change of convergence is performed satisfactorily. Normally, a prompt and smooth convergence movement from distance fixation to near is seen. There are four types of abnormal response which may be observed:

(a) Over-convergence; this may be followed by a corrective movement. This is not significant in the context of convergence insufficiency.
(b) Versional movement: both eyes move an equal amount to allow the dominant eye to take up fixation while the other diverges.
(c) Slow or hesitant movement.
(d) No movement of either eye or of only one eye.

The last three of these responses indicate a failure of normal convergence, and it is likely that there will be trouble in maintaining convergence for near vision. Clearly, all clinical tests need to be completed in a short time, but what is important to the patient is whether symptoms will arise during longer periods of reading and close work. However, if the patient has a near point of convergence of 10–15 cm, and the jump convergence is normal, it is unlikely that there will be symptoms. Failure on the jump convergence test occurs more often than a poor near point, and appears to be associated with symptoms more frequently (Pickwell and Hampshire, 1981a). Some patients can perform well on the near point test by exercising an unusual amount of effort, but cannot maintain this degree of convergence for sustained near vision. The jump convergence test seems the more useful clinical test, but both should be included in routine examination of convergence.

(3) *Heterophoria tests for near vision*, which usually show compensated exophoria. In about one-third of the patients with convergence insufficiency there is decompensated exophoria for near vision (Pickwell and Hampshire, 1981a). This is more likely to occur in the very elderly patient. Fixation disparity tests for near vision show suppression of one of the monocular markers in about one-fifth of the convergence insufficiency cases. In the absence of a squint, this suppression for near vision can be taken as a possible indication of the presence of convergence inadequacy.

(4) *Amplitude of accommodation*, which is low with some patients. These cases of convergence and accommodation insufficiency are distinguished from ophthalmoplegia (see Chapter 16), as the latter condition has a sudden onset of symptoms. Convergence insufficiency with accommodation insufficiency usually starts to give trouble in the teenage years, and sometimes improves after several years. The AC/A ratio is very low in these cases.

Management

Treatment of convergence insufficiency is usually by orthoptic procedures and is nearly always successful, even with older patients. The management will be considered under the five general headings given in Chapter 4. on the basic principles of management.

REMOVAL OF CAUSE OF DECOMPENSATION

The factors that create decompensation of heterophoria may also aggravate convergence insufficiency, so that thought should be given to the working conditions, to the general health and to the general well-being of the patient.

REFRACTIVE CORRECTION

A spectacle correction should be given where necessary. When convergence insufficiency is combined with accommodative insufficiency in teenage patients, it is usually necessary to give a reading addition. The power is decided on the basis of allowing the patient to use about two-thirds of the amplitude of accommodation for the normal near working distances, the rest being made up by the reading addition. Base-in prism may also help in these particular cases. The prism power can be determined by giving the weakest prism which will allow the patient to show prompt and smooth convergence on the jump convergence test. These patients seem to take a long time to settle to any prescription given. Such cases of convergence and accommodative insufficiency do not respond to orthoptic treatment, described below, for the more usual convergence insufficiency pattern. Early teenage patients with previously uncorrected myopia may find the refraction correction relieves the convergence insufficiency.

ORTHOPTIC TREATMENT

'Pencil-to-nose' type exercises are usually given, and prove quite successful for convergence insufficiency. The patient looks at the tip of a pencil held at about arm's length and is asked to see it singly while some other object further away is seen in physiological diplopia. The pencil is then slowly moved towards the eyes while it is maintained singly for as long as possible. The procedure is repeated until the pencil can be approached closer than 10 cm before doubling occurs. The physiological diplopia of a more distant object is maintained as a check on suppression. Sometimes preliminary exercises for suppression are required before the pencil-to-nose exercises.

Another type of exercise which can also be useful in convergence problems is the physiological diplopia exercise for vergence co-ordination, which is described for divergence weakness type of esophoria in the previous chapter. In cases of convergence insufficiency, the nearer object is held at 40 cm from the eyes in the first place, but gradually moved closer as the patient is able to alternate between near fixation with uncrossed physiological diplopia and distance fixation with crossed diplopia. By this procedure, the patient is encouraged to perform the jump convergence test, with the nearer fixation object starting at 40 cm and gradually moving closer to the eyes to the 15 cm position.

Patients will usually be able to teach themselves to develop a near point of convergence of less than 10 cm, and to perform the jump convergence test quite quickly - usually in several weeks. The exercise should be continued for 2 weeks after this. If this is not done, the convergence insufficiency problem may recur after a short time. Indeed, with some patients it may be necessary to repeat the exercises at intervals of a few months to maintain adequate convergence. However, if the convergence insufficiency does recur after a few months, more thought should be given to the possibility of aggravating factors such as poor general health or inadequate lighting, etc.

RELIEVING PRISMS

These are not appropriate to convergence insufficiency, except when it is combined with accommodative insufficiency, as described above.

REFERRAL

Usually, convergence insufficiency is treated by orthoptic exercises and does not require referral. Where primary spasm of convergence is suspected, or where it is combined with the signs of a primary pathological cause, the patient will require medical investigation; for example, where it appears with other indications of thyroid problems – Moebius's sign (see Chapter 16 for thyrotoxicosis).

References

BREININ, G. N. (1957). The nature of vergence revealed by electromyography, Part III. *Archives of Ophthalmology*, **58,** 623–635

BURIAN, H. M. and VON NOORDEN, G. K. (1974). *Binocular Vision and Ocular Motility*. Mosby, St. Louis, p. 305

DUANE, A. (1897). A new classification of the motor anomalies of the eye. *Annals of Ophthalmology*, **6,** 250

EUSTACE, P., WESTON, E. and DRUBY, D. J. (1973). The effect of illumination on intermittent divergent squint of the divergence excess type. *Transactions of the Ophthalmological Society of Great Britain,* **93,** 559–590

FREIER, B. and PICKWELL, L. D. (1983). Physiological exophoria. *Ophthalmic and Physiological Optics*, **3**(3), 267 272

GRAEFE, A. VON (1862). Quoted in Burian and von Noorden (see above), p. 395

LONDON, R. F. and WICK, B. (1987). Vertical fixation disparity correction: effect on the horizontal forced-vergence fixation disparity curve. *American Journal of Optometry,* **64**(9), 653–655

LYLE, T. K. and WYBAR, K. C. (1967). *Practical Orthoptics in the Treatment of Squint*. Lewis, London, p. 428

PICKWELL, L. D. (1979). Prevalence and management of divergence excess. *American Journal of Optometry*, **56**(2), 78–81

PICKWELL, L. D. (1985). The increase in convergence inadequacy with age. *Ophthalmic and Physiological Optics,* **5**(3), 347–348

PICKWELL, L. D. and HAMPSHIRE, R. (1981a). The significance of inadequate convergence. *Ophthalmic and Physiological Optics*, **1,** 13–18

PICKWELL, L. D. and HAMPSHIRE, R. (1981b). Jump convergence test in strabismus. *Ophthalmic and Physiological Optics*, **1,** 123–124

PICKWELL, L. D. and HAMPSHIRE, R. (1984). Convergence insufficiency in patients taking medicines. *Ophthalmic and Physiological Optics,* **4** (2), 151–154

PICKWELL, L. D., VIGGARS, M. A. and JENKINS, T. C. A. (1986). Convergence insufficiency in a rural population. *Ophthalmic and Physiological Optics,* **6**(3), 339–340

7

Hyperphoria

Hyperphoria is a potential deviation of one eye upwards which becomes an actual deviation when the two eyes are dissociated and which recovers when the dissociating factors are removed. In hypophoria, the deviation is downwards, and as hypophoria of one eye may be regarded as the same as hyperphoria of the other, the term 'hypophoria' is not in general use: note that right hyperphoria is the same as left hypophoria. Occasionaliy, vertical heterophoria occurs in one eye only, which is usually found to be amblyopic.

Secondary hyperphoria

Aetiology

Hyperphoria is often present as a secondary condition, and the primary causes should be considered before treating the hyperphoria. It may be secondary to the following.

HORIZONTAL HETEROPHORIA

High degrees of comitant esophoria or exophoria are often accompanied by a small vertical component. In these cases, the treatment will be that which is appropriate to the primary condition, but prism relief of the hyperphoria may help.

INCOMITANT DEVIATIONS

Paretic conditions involving the elevator or depressor muscles may begin as hyperphoria and develop later into a squint. It is important that this early sign of pathology should be detected. The sudden onset of intermittent vertical diplopia and other symptoms, and the incomitant nature of the heterophoria, are the main diagnostic features. Congenital incomitant deviations are also accompanied by a vertical element, but symptoms are usually absent.

TILTED SPECTACLES

If spectacles are incorrectly fitted or the frame becomes bent, a vertical prism element may be introduced which will initially show as hyperphoria. Usually, the patient will adapt quite quickly to this abnormal prism and the hyperphoria will no longer be apparent. When this occurs, hyperphoria will be present when the glasses are removed or the spectacle frame straightened. This will disappear after a few days. Corrections for anisometropia may also produce hyperphoria when the eyes are not looking through the optical centres. Again, adaptation to this variable prismatic effect will usually occur after a few days of using the anisometropic correction, but difficulties can arise if a correction for marked anisometropia is given in cases where no glasses have been worn before (see also Chapter 9).

A spectacle correction which has not been correctly balanced between the two eyes may also cause hyperphoria. The same applies to uncorrected anisometropia.

Primary hyperphoria

Primary hyperphoria is usually considered to be largely due to slight anatomical misalignments of the eyes and/or orbits or muscle insertions for which there is a physiological compensation. Usually, this type of hyperphoria is less than 3^{Δ}, and it seldom causes symptoms. It has been shown that about 98% of symptom-free people will show some degree of hyperphoria after a period of prolonged occlusion of one eye, but this disappears after a few hours when the binocular vision is restored (Duke-Elder, 1973). Vertical heterophoria is not associated with the convergence system in the way that applies to horizontal heterophoria, and this further suggests that anatomical factors play a larger part in its aetiology.

However, decompensation can occur in hyperphoria due to stress on the visual system or on the general well-being of the patient (see Chapter 1).

Investigation

A routine eye examination should be carried out; the following points may be particularly useful in hyperphoria:

(1) *Symptoms*, which can sometimes be very marked in hyperphoria, even where the degree of the heterophoria is low. They occur more frequently in middle age. Frontal headache, ocular discomfort or pain and blephritis are the most common symptoms. Sometimes there is a head tilt, and other patients may report that vision is more comfortable if one eye is closed or occluded.
(2) *Motility test* for incomitancy, which should always be undertaken with objective observation of the eyes and also noting the subjective response of the patient reporting any incomitant diplopia (see Chapter 2 for the routine, and Chapter 16 for the diagnosis of incomitant deviations).
(3) *Refraction*, which should give particular attention to the binocular balance of the spherical error between the two eyes. An unbalanced correction can sometimes be the cause of hyperphoria. The balancing can be done by near-fixation retinoscopy or subjectively by an infinity balance method.
(4) *Compensation assessment*, which should be made as described in Chapter 3. The cover test, infinity balance test and fixation disparity tests will prove useful in making this assessment for hyperphoria.

Management

REMOVAL OF CAUSE OF DECOMPENSATION

Care must be taken to explore the visual working conditions and any stress or ill-health that may be the cause of the decompensation. These should receive attention before other aspects of management.

REFRACTIVE CORRECTION

In many cases, the provision of a correction for previously uncorrected refractive error will alleviate the hyperphoria without any other treatment. Balancing the refractive correction is very important in hyperphoria and can be done by near-fixation retinoscopy and further checked subjectively by an infinity balance test or the Mallett fixation disparity unit. These later tests also are very useful for prescribing any prism relief which is sometimes required.

Near-fixation retinoscopy (not dynamic retinoscopy) is a useful method of checking the spherical balance between the two eyes (Hodd, 1951). Static retinoscopy is carried out with distance fixation in the usual way. The patient is then asked to look at a target on or in the plane of the retinoscope. The instrument is held at the normal distance from the patient's eyes for static retinoscopy (66 cm) and not at the near-vision distance. With the static refraction and the 'working distance' lenses in place, the fixation target will be conjugate with the patient's retina and there will be little stimulus to accommodation. Most patients do not accommodate, as the degree of convergence and proximal stimulus is not marked. Under these conditions, the retinoscope light can be passed over each of the two eyes in very quick succession, and neutralization obtained by small spherical adjustments in both eyes almost simultaneously.

The infinity balance test or septum test (see Chapter 3) is particularly useful in hyperphoria. It also illustrates very clearly the importance of spherical balance in many hyperphoria cases. The septum is set up so that the patient can see the letter F with the right eye and L with the left. The questions are asked, 'Are both letters seen and are they equally clear and level, or is one letter clearer or higher than the other?' If both letters are seen, there is no marked suppression. If one is clearer or higher than the other, a +0.25 D sphere is held before the less clear eye to see if it blurs further. If it equalizes the acuities, it is incorporated in the prescription. If it blurs, it is tried before the other eye to obtain balance. If the +0.25 D sphere blurs both eyes, then a −0.25 D sphere is tried.

With many cases of vertical misalignment of the letters initially, the letters are levelled by the balancing of the spherical part of the prescription. If this does not occur, the weakest vertical prism is found which will level the letters. This prism may be incorporated into the prescription.

If the patient is slightly amblyopic in one eye, the spherical balance can be found by the use of the near-fixation retinoscopy method described above, or by a subjective bichromatic test such as the Freeman binocular bichromatic test (see *Figure 3.2*. This enables the correcting sphere to be found in both eyes simultaneously, by balancing the clarity of the circles on the red ground with those on the green – both seen on one side of the septum with the right eye, and both seen simultaneously on the other side of the septum with the left eye. In this case, it is a matter of balancing the red and green on each side of the septum, and not comparing the right eye with the left.

In the case of marked anisometropia where no previous correction has been worn, a partial correction of the more hyperopic eye may prevent disturbance by vertical prismatic effects when the patient is not looking through the optical centres of the lenses. The correction is reduced in the more hyperopic eye until the vertical heterophoria is compensated when looking through the lenses a little above or below the optical centres. This can be judged by Turville's 'nodding test'. The infinity balance septum is used and the patient asked to raise and lower his head in a slight nodding motion until the reduction of the sphere does not create a change of level in the two letters. A similar method can be used by nodding while observing the Mallett fixation disparity test. This correction may be increased to a fuller prescription with subsequent glasses (see also Chapter 9).

ORTHOPTIC TREATMENT

Orthoptic exercises to improve the vertical prism vergences very seldom prove successful, and do not seem to help in making the hyperphoria compensated.

When the hyperphoria is associated with horizontal heterophoria, orthoptic exercises to increase the horizontal prism vergences will often result in the vertical heterophoria becoming compensated.

RELIEVING PRISMS

Most primary hyperphoria can be readily relieved by small vertical prisms. As explained above, the smallest prism that will level the infinity balance test letters or that will neutralize the fixation disparity with a Mallett unit can be prescribed. Such vertical prism relief may also help any decompensated horizontal heterophoria (see Chapter 6).

REFERRAL

Incomitant hyperphoria with intermittent diplopia of recent onset indicates the need for medical investigation. When there is a high degree of hyperphoria and congenital incomitancy which gives rise to intolerable symptoms, surgical relief is sometimes considered. Medical advice should be sought.

Dissociated vertical deviation

This is a comparatively unusual anomaly which is also known as 'alternating sursumduction'. Although it could be mistaken for hyperphoria, the clinical appearance is not the same. It is usually seen during the cover test. When one eye is covered with an occluder or a dark filter, it slowly deviates upwards possibly as much as 20°. This differs from hyperphoria in that, whichever eye is covered, there is an *upward* movement of the eye behind the cover. When the cover is removed, the eye slowly recovers to the fixation position. The upward movement is not always equal in the two eyes, and sometimes it can be absent in one eye giving the appearance of a 'unilateral hyperphoria'. In all cases, if a neutral density filter bar is placed before the uncovered eye and the density of the filter increased, the eye under the cover will slowly move down; when the density of filter is reduced, the covered eye moves slowly up again – the Bielschowsky test.

Dissociated vertical deviation is often associated with convergent squint and there is sometimes nystagmus of the deviated eye during the cover test. Even when there is no squint or other reason to suspect an inferior oblique palsy, there is sometimes a cyclorotation of the occluded eye (Burian and von Noorden, 1974).

The aetiology of this condition is obscure, When it exists without any other deviation or anomaly, there are usually no symptoms and no independent treatment is required. If it exists with other conditions, treatment appropriate to the primary condition can be considered. Occasionally, patients with dissociated vertical deviation complain that one eye deviates spontaneously and that this is noticed by other people. However, there seems to be no appropriate treatment (Burian and von Noorden, 1974).

Cyclophoria

It is doubtful if cyclophoria exists as a primary condition not associated with incomitant deviations. Kertesz and Jones (1970) showed by an objective means that cyclofusion has no motor component. There seems to be no evidence of the diagnosis of primary cyclophoria, although many authorities give methods for its detection (Duke-Elder, 1973).

References

BURIAN, H. and VON NOORDEN, G. K. (1974). *Binocular Vision and Ocular Motility*. Mosby, St. Louis, p. 320

DUKE-ELDER, SIR STEWART (1973). *System of Ophthalmology*, vol. VI, *Ocular Motility and Strabismus*. Kimpton, London, p. 551

HODD, F. A. B. (1951). The measurement of spherical refraction by retinoscopy. *Transactions of the International Congress of the British Optical Association*, pp. 191–231

KERTESZ, A. E. and JONES, R. W. (1970). Human cyclofusional response. *Vision Research*, **10,** 891–896

8

Orthoptic exercises for heterophoria

The general outlines to be followed by orthoptic treatment in particular binocular anomalies are given in the preceding chapters which deal with the anomalies. This chapter gives details of particular exercises which may be fitted into the aims outlined. For example, the treatment of central suppression is appropriate to several different anomalies. The details of a number of exercises for the treatment of suppression are given below rather than repeating them in several of the previous chapters.

The general principles of orthoptic treatment and the factors to be considered in the selection of patients are described in Chapter 4.

Exercises in this chapter will be considered under three main headings: (1) exercises for the treatment of central suppression; (2) development of prism vergences and relative accommodation; (3) general co-ordination and convergence exercises.

Exercises for treatment of central suppression

In heterophoria, suppression is mostly confined to a small area within the field of the macula and is usually intermittent. Only where there is a long-standing intermittent squint, as in divergence excess, will a larger suppression area be present. Where suppression is demonstrated, it is treated first or at the same time as any vergence treatment. All or some of the following exercises may be appropriate.

Stereoscope cards

Several stereoscope cards have been designed for the treatment of suppression in heterophoria. These usually consist of 'fusion' cards, in which most of the design is common to both eyes, but some of the detail is presented to one eye only. The patient is asked to look at the fused design and ensure that the part of the total picture presented only to the eye with a tendency to suppress is seen and is retained without intermittently disappearing. Examples of this type of card are shown in *Figure 8.1*, which illustrates several of the F series in the Bradford Set of Stereoscope Cards. Each card contains a printed passage in which the letters are

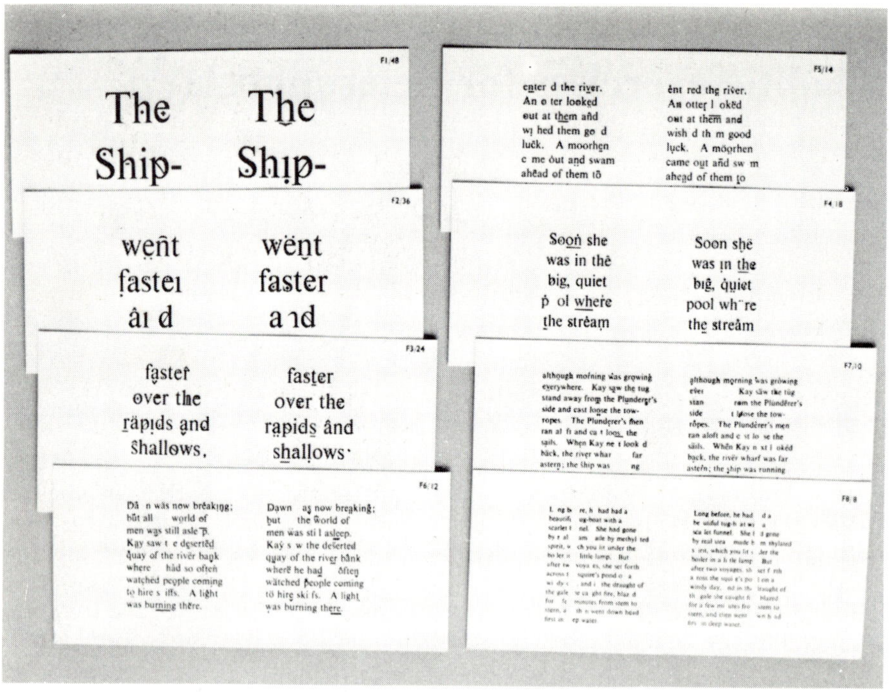

Figure 8.1. Bradford F series stereoscope cards, for the treatment of central suppression

interrupted by the addition of dots, marks, crosses, lines, etc., before one eye, or in which some of the letters are missing before one eye. The patient needs to overcome the suppression in order to see all the monocular additions or omissions. Each card is printed in a different size of type, from N48 down to N6. Obviously, the smaller the print, the more difficult it becomes to overcome the suppression. The patient starts with the larger print cards and works through to the limit of the acuity.

Other cases are illustrated (G series) in which there is a binocularly seen black frame to assist in maintaining fusion. In this series, some of the letters are printed in red, and the exercise can be made more difficult by the use of a red filter before one eye. In the L series, the principle is similar, but a pictorial design is incorporated (see *Figure 8.2*).

These cards can be used in any suitable stereoscope. If an exercise is required for a binocular anomaly for near vision, the prism stereoscope (*Figure 8.2*) can be used, or a Holmes stereoscope (see *Figure 8.9*), adjusted for a near image. Where the anomaly is present for distance vision, a Holmes stereoscope in the infinity adjustment, i.e. a card at the focal length of the lenses, is used.

Physiological diplopia

There are a number of ways in which the use of physiological diplopia can be useful in the treatment of heterophoria. First, it should be demonstrated that the patient can appreciate physiological diplopia using two fairly large and obvious objects as targets; for example two pencils or ball-point pens of different colours. The method

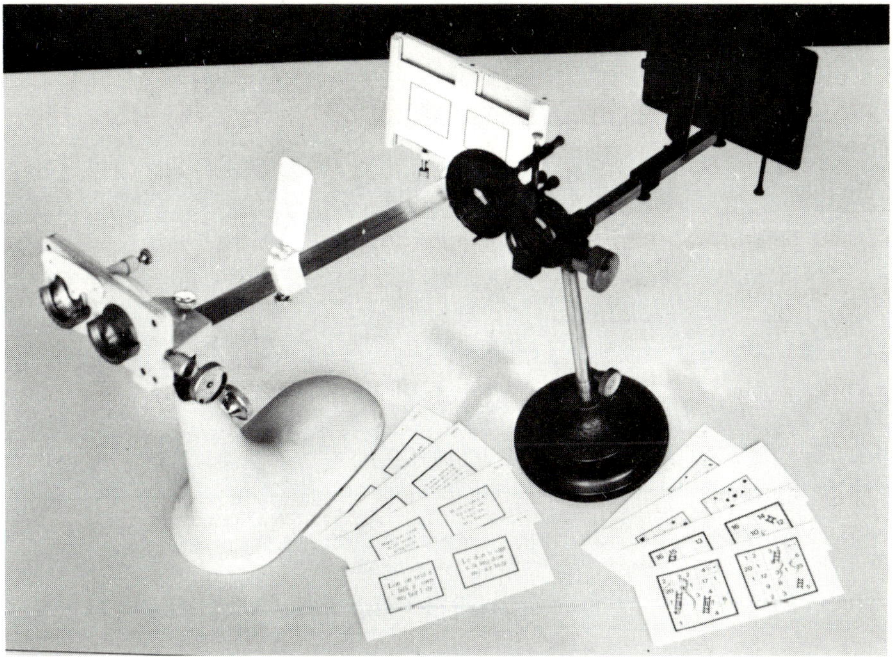

Figure 8.2. Two models of the variable prism stereoscope with the Bradford stereoscope cards, G and L series, for the treatment of central suppression – pictorial design

of demonstrating this is shown in (*Figure 8.3*). The demonstration should include the patient fixing the nearer pencil and noticing the far pencil in uncrossed physiological diplopia, and then fixing the far pencil and observing the near one in crossed diplopia. Difficulty in seeing both the diplopic images indicates a fairly gross degree of suppression, which is usually overcome quite quickly in heterophoria. However, many patients may have difficulty in alternating between uncrossed and crossed diplopia. In these cases, it is useful to ask the patient to practise doing this alternation as an exercise; this is described later in the third section of this chapter.

When the patient has appreciated physiological diplopia with the pencils, macular suppression can be treated by using thinner targets such as a thin knitting needle or a straightened length (about 15 cm) of wire. This is interposed between the eyes and a page of print (see *Figure 8.4*). This is the *wire reading* method. Initially, it is placed at the mid-distance from the eyes to the page, so that it is seen in physiological diplopia with two images apparently separated by 1 or 2 cm.

The patient is asked to read the page, slowly moving the wire along to keep the word being read mid-way between the two diplopic images and being conscious of both images all the time. When this is done, the wire is moved slightly nearer to the page so that its images appear closer together and more into the central suppression area. The patient should be asked to practise this exercise for several 10-minute periods each day for one or two weeks (Earnshaw, 1960). In the case of children, the exercise needs to be supervised by a parent to ensure that they do not forget to maintain a check that both diplopic images are there, otherwise interest in the book may absorb all their attention.

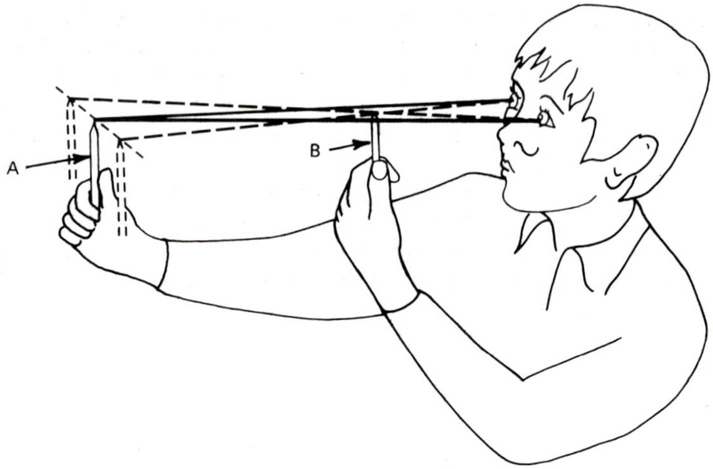

Figure 8.3. Physiological diplopia: the patient fixes the further pencil A and notices that the nearer pencil B is seen in crossed physiological diplopia – the right eye's image on the left and the left eye's image on the right. A change of fixation to the nearer pencil should result in the farther one being seen in uncrossed physiological diplopia. For details of exercises, see text

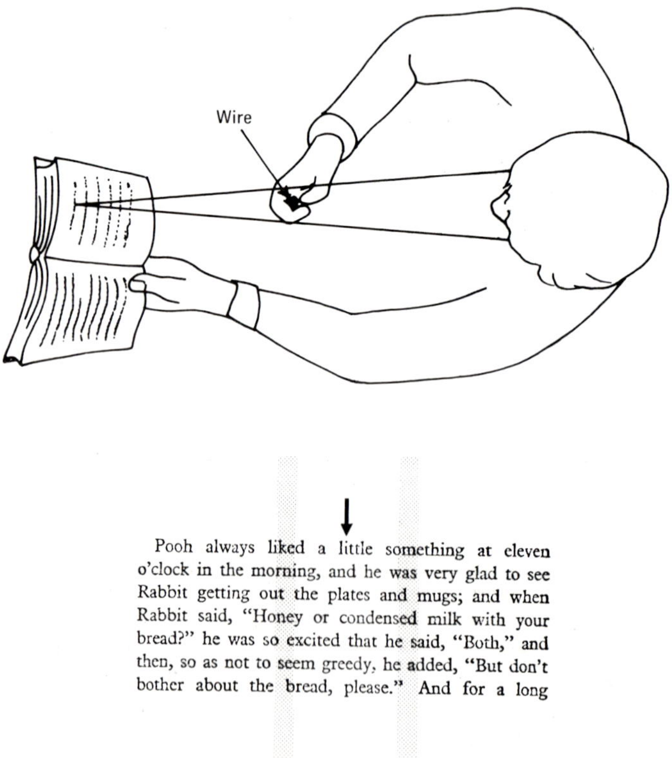

Figure 8.4. Wire reading: a thin rod or length of wire is held on the median line between the printed page and the eyes. When fixing a letter on the page, the wire is seen in uncrossed physiological diplopia (see lower diagram) unless there is suppression. As the patient reads, the wire is moved across the page to maintain the two images at equal distance on each side of the point of fixation

Bar reading is a further extension of this exercise (see *Figure 8.5*). In this case, the patient uses a thicker object; a pencil is appropriate, but an even more thick object can be used. If a pencil is interposed between the eyes and the book, it should be about one-third of the distance from the eyes. This will ensure that it acts like a septum, occluding a vertical strip of the print from each eye. In this exercise, the pencil is held still on the median line, and is not moved along the line as in the previous method. As the patient's eyes cross the page during reading, the beginning of the line is seen by both eyes. There is then a strip occluded from the right eye by the pencil, but visible to the left if there is no suppression. Then there is a strip of the page seen by both eyes before the pencil occludes the left eye. The end of each line of print may be seen by both eyes.

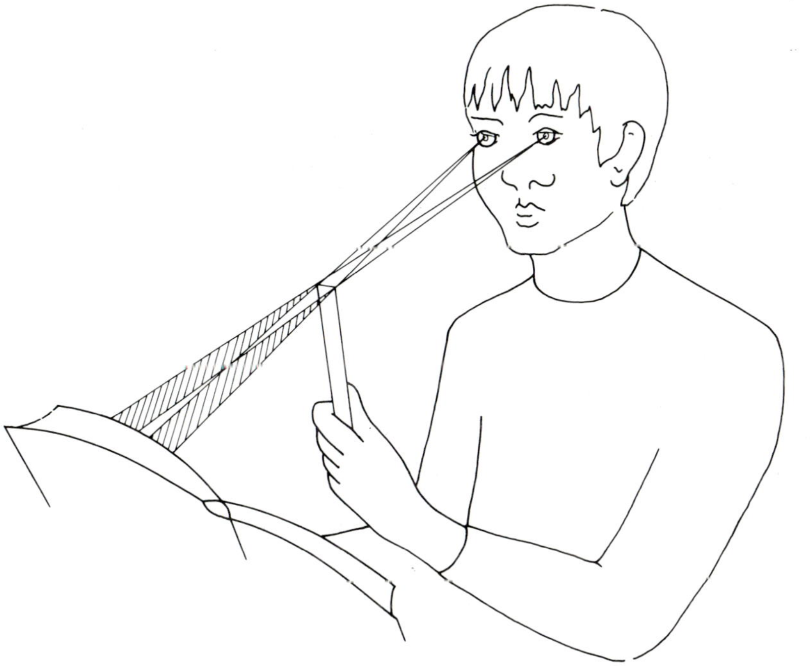

Figure 8.5. Bar reading: a slightly wider septum is held a little closer than mid-way between the page and the eyes. It is kept still on the median line so that it occludes a different part of the page from each eye. The patient must use both eyes to be able to read across the page

Unless there is suppression, the patient should be able to read across the page without being aware of the pencil occluding either eye. At first, the patient may have to make a conscious effort to 'see through' the pencil in the position where it occludes the dominant eye. It is important that during the exercise the head is held quite still. If the patient experiences difficulty in the exercise, small movements of the head will be noted as he or she tries to look round the pencil. A parent or friend may need to watch that this does not happen.

If the suppression is present mainly for distance vision, the *septum test* (see *Figure 8.6*) can be modified to provide an exercise. The patient holds a finger or other object of about the same width, 10–20 cm from the eyes, while looking across the room or out of a window for distance vision. It is noticed that the 'septum'

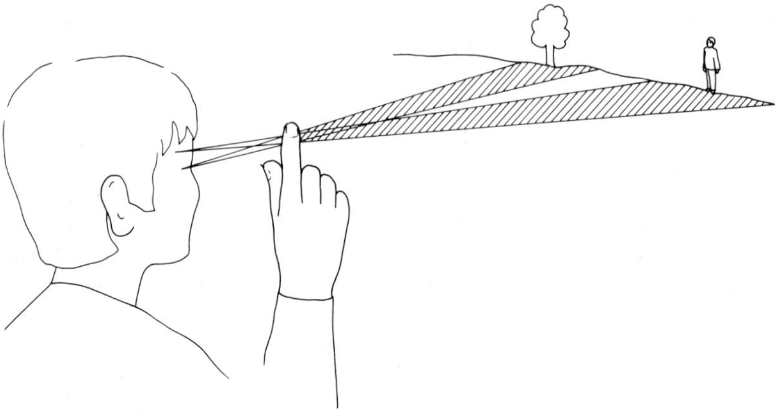

Figure 8.6. A septum for exercising simultaneous vision for distance vision. The finger (or a septum) is held about 10 cm from the eyes while the patient looks at a distant scene. The patient should be aware of physiological diplopia of the finger and that both images are apparently transparent; that is, an object can be seen 'through' each finger, e.g. the tree and the man. The patient alternates fixation from one subject to the other, pausing at each to ensure that both objects and images of the finger are still visible

occludes objects in the visual field from each eye. The patient is asked to identify these objects by closing each eye in turn or by occluding each with the other hand, e.g. the tree and the man in *Figure 8.6*. Then, with both eyes open, he or she is asked to look first at one of the objects and then at the other, alternating between the two. The head and hand must be kept quite still during this, and the patient is asked to concentrate on seeing 'through' the finger each time there is a tendency to

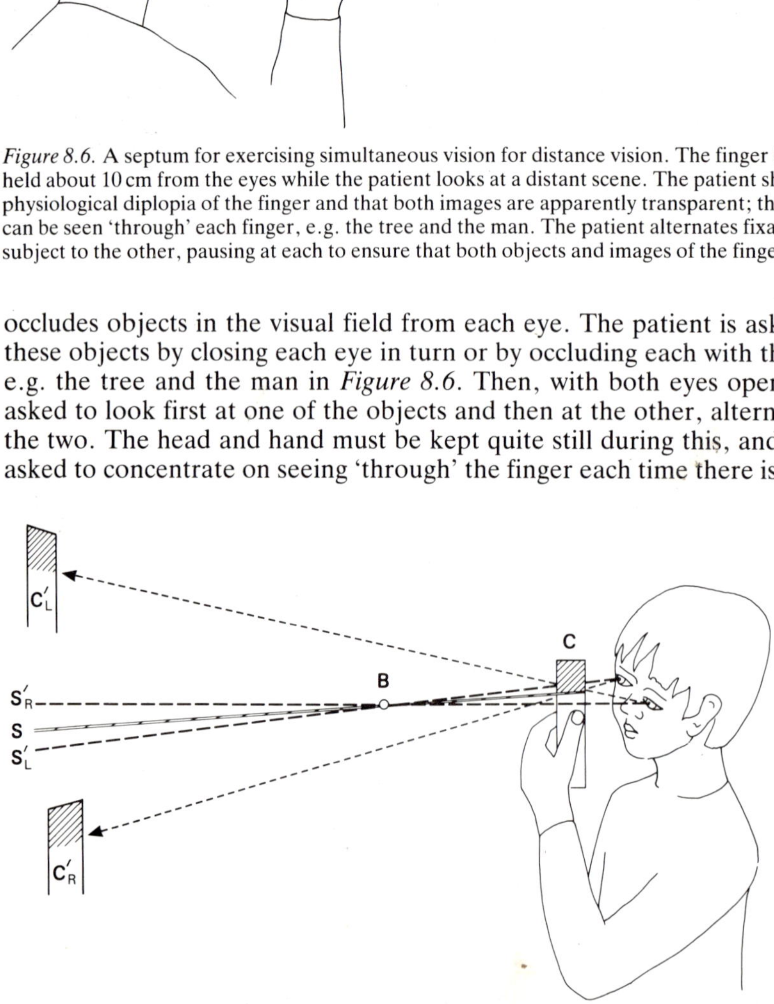

Figure 8.7. Bead-on-string exercise: the patient holds a card, C, close to the nose. A length of string, SBC, tied to the card and to some more distant object, stretches horizontally. A bead, B, acts as a fixation object. The patient, fixing the bead, should see the card in crossed physiological diplopia: if it is a different colour on each side, it helps identification of the crossed diplopia. The string will be seen in increasing uncrossed diplopia beyond the fixation point, S'_R and S'_L, and in increasing crossed diplopia between the fixation bead and the eyes; that is, the string should appear as two strings crossing through the bead. In suppression, part of the cross will not be seen. For details of the exercise, see text

suppress. The exercise can be demonstrated in the consulting room using a distance of 6 m and two objects about 75 cm apart: the finger is moved nearer to the eyes or further away to obtain the best position.

The *bead-on-string* exercise can be used to combine near and distance vision exercises. This has been used very successfully in the Bradford University clinics for many years (Pickwell, 1971; 1979). A length of string is tied at one end to a suitable object several metres from the patient, and the near end held close to the nose so that the patient looks down the length of the string (see *Figure 8.7*). A piece of card with a different colour patch on each side is seen in crossed physiological diplopia to check for gross suppression. A bead, or small hexagonal metal nut, is threaded on the string and serves as a movable fixation target. The string should be seen in continuous physiological diplopia, with the 'two strings' appearing to cross at the fixation, i.e. through the bead or nut. Any suppression is indicated by the lack of seeing part of one of the two strings; closer than fixation in the case of exophoria, and beyond fixation in esophoria. The fixation bead or nut can be moved along the string to check for suppression at all distances. With a little practice the patient can move fixation along the string without having to move the bead or nut, and can maintain a continuous check on suppression at all distances.

Note that this procedure does not exercise relative convergence, as the accommodation and convergence are changed together. It may, however, assist in heterophoria cases where the patient has difficulty in appreciating physiological diplopia correctly – this is further developed later in the chapter.

Red and green filters

If the eyes are dissociated by placing before one eye a red filter and before the other a green one, while the patient looks at a small spot of light, any suppression will show as an absence of one colour. Normal patients will see one light which is a mixture of red and green in retinal rivalry. In unstable heterophoria, two lights may be seen and where there is suppression one of these may be present only intermittently. A prism of 6^{Δ}, base downwards before one eye, will produce vertical diplopia, and suppression is more easily overcome.

In this exercise, the prism is rotated slowly toward the base direction in which it relieves the heterophoria; base-in for exophoria or base-out for esophoria. The patient will see the two lights rotate round each other and move closer together as they become level and the prism relieves the phoria. As the images move into the central macular suppression area, one colour will disappear. The prism base–apex line is turned back towards its original base-down position and the patient tries to see the missing colour (Humphriss, 1953). The patient can have red and green filters and a prism on loan to practise this at home. This exercise is particularly useful in divergence excess cases.

Development of prism vergences and relative accommodation

Orthoptic exercises seldom seem to change the magnitude of the heterophoria, and where there is a reduction in degree this seems to be temporary only. However, it is possible to increase the prism vergence and also the relative accommodation, and this usually results in making the heterophoria compensated so that the patient has no symptoms. Prism vergence (fusional reserve or relative convergence) exercises may be combined with the development of relative accommodation. The aim of the exercise appropriate to each kind of anomaly has been described in the previous chapters for each condition, but the general principles can be summarized as follows:

(1) In esophoric conditions – develop *base-in* prism vergence and/or positive relative accommodation.
(2) In exophoric conditions – develop *base-out* prism vergence and/or negative relative accommodation.

In general, the object of this type of exercise is to exert the prism vergence while keeping the accommodation unchanged: or, the other way round, induce changes in the accommodation while maintaining fixed convergence. Some methods exercise both, but one function is changed in excess of the other. The intention is to strengthen and increase the function which opposes the troublesome heterophoria, and to extend the range, or to 'loosen up', the accommodation–convergence relationship.

Variable prism devices

These devices are the simplest and most direct method of exercising the prism vergence (or fusional reserve). A variable prism device, such as a rotary prism, prism bar or the prisms of a variable prism stereoscope, is used in the same way as described for the measurement of prism vergences in Chapter 3. The patient looks at letters small enough to require precise convergence and accommodation while the power of the prism is gradually increased. The patient is asked to maintain clear single vision as long as possible, but when blurring or doubling occurs, the prism power is reduced and the patient asked to recover clear single vision as soon as possible. The procedure is repeated for periods of about 5 minutes. The exercise is carried out for near vision or distance vision, or both, as the patient's difficulties suggest is appropriate.

If a variable stereoscope is used for distance vision, the card holder is removed and the patient looks across the room. For near vision, this instrument can be used either with a single line of letters in the card holder and the septum removed, or using a stereoscope card with separate right and left eye pictures and with the septum in place. In the latter case, 9^{Δ} out in each eye will be required. The stereoscope cards appropriate for this should have the majority of the picture common to both eyes so that 'fusion' can take place, but have small parts of each eye's picture presented to only one eye to act as 'control marks'. In those cases where suppression is particularly marked, this type of card should be used in the early stages of treatment. Note that in all cases the patient should be asked to report that doubling has been observed, in the sense that the target is seen to break into two and the images drift apart. In some cases, double vision may not occur until one of the images has moved outside a fairly large retinal suppression area. In these cases, the target is not seen to double but a second peripheral image suddenly appears; this is most likely in divergence excess exophoria.

Holmes stereoscope

The optics principle of this instrument is summarized in *Figure 8.8*, and examples of the instruments are illustrated in *Figure 8.9*, which also shows examples of suitable

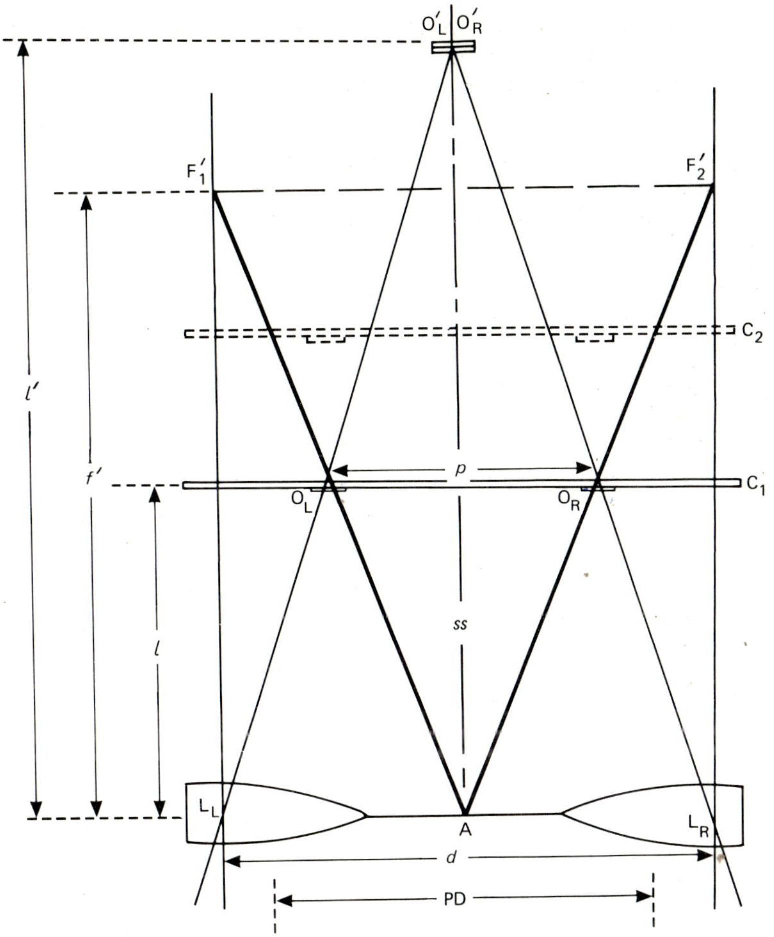

Figure 8.8. The principle of the Holmes stereoscope. Two lenses, L_R and L_L, are separated by a distance, *d*, which is greater that the patient's pupillary distance, so that a base-out prism effect is produced. A septum at *ss* prevents the right eye from seeing the left image, and the left eye from seeing the right image. The pictures, O_R and O_L, on the card C_1, are held at a distance, *l*. If these pictures are separated by a distance, *p*, such that they lie on the two lines joining the focal points of the lenses, F'_1 and F'_2, with the mid-point between the lenses, A (the 'orthophoria' lines), the images of the pictures, O'_L and O'_R, will coincide on the mid-line at a distance, *l′*. The eyes should then have to exert accommodation and convergence in the normal relationship for looking at an object at *l′* (ignoring proximal convergence). If the pictures lie outside the orthophoria lines, forced divergence will be required for single vision. Such forced divergence, which is required as an exercise in esophoric conditions, can be achieved by either increasing the picture separation, *p*, or by decreasing the card distance, *l*. Similarly, the forced convergence required in exercises for exophoric conditions can be produced by decreasing the picture separation or by increasing the card distance; e.g. moving the card to C_2 (after Lyle and Wybar, 1967)

designs of cards for developing vergences and relative accommodation. It will be seen from *Figure 8.8* that a lens stereoscope can be considered to have two 'orthophoria lines' (Asher and Law, 1952) from the focal point of each of the lenses to a point mid-way between the lenses themselves. In most stereoscopes, these are purely imaginary lines, but are useful in deciding which exercise is appropriate to esophoria or to exophoria. If the two pictures on the stereoscope card are of such a

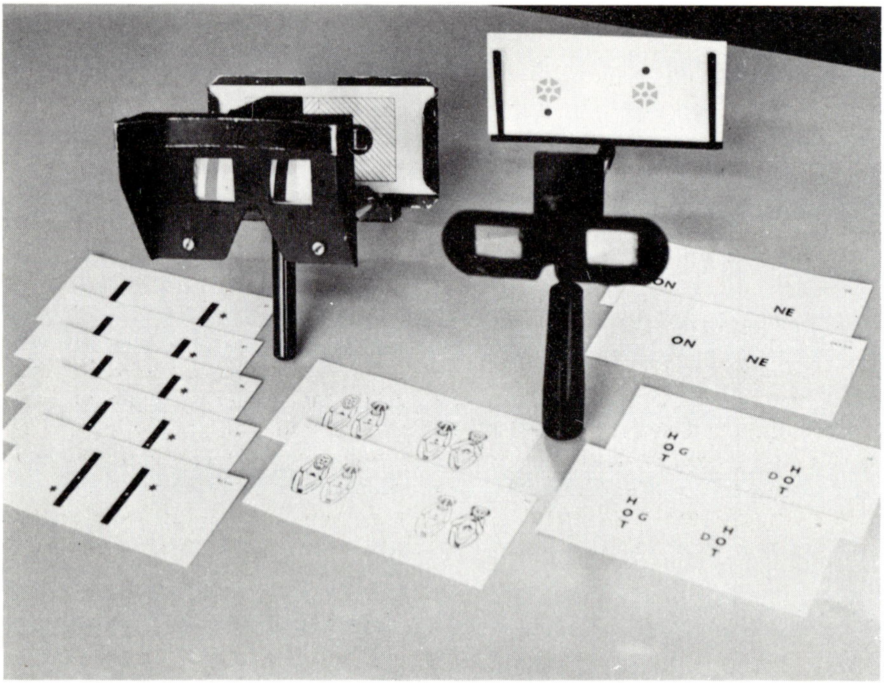

Figure 8.9. Two models of the Holmes stereoscope with Bradford stereoscope cards: the C series 'ruby' card is in the right-hand stereoscope; B series, bar and star design; M series, three wise monkeys; D series, ON NE Wells cards; E series, stereoscopic design HOT DOG. Each of these series is available in increasing picture separations for exercising forced vergence training

separation and at such a distance that they fall one on each of these orthophoria lines, their images will coincide with each other on the mid-line of the instrument. This will mean that, ignoring any proximal convergence, the eyes will have to converge and accommodate according to the normal accommodation–convergence relationship for the particular distance of the images. To use a card with a greater picture separation, but at the same card distance, would require the eyes to diverge in order to 'fuse', and a card with less picture separation would induce convergence. No change in accommodation would be required.

The diagram in *Figure 8.8* also shows that if the card distance is increased without changing the separation of the pictures, i.e. the card holder is drawn away from the patient's eyes, the picture separation will now be narrow for the new card distance and therefore convergence will be required to maintain 'fusion'. In this new position, the card's picture will lie inside the orthophoria lines. At the same time, the image distance will have increased, so that less accommodation will be required. This means that when the card distance is increased, convergence and negative relative accommodation will be exercised which will help patients with exophoric conditions. In summary, when using the Holmes strereoscope:

(1) In esophoric conditions – use cards of increasing picture separation and/or move the card holder *towards* the patient's eyes.
(2) In exophoric conditions – use cards of decreasing picture separation and/or move the card holder *away from* the patient's eyes.

Over the years, a number of cards have been designed for this type of exercise, of which the Bradford Set of Stereoscope Cards is typical. This set provides several suitable designs. Some of these are illustrated in *Figure 8.9*, which shows cards appropriate at various stages of treatment and of patient age range. The B series has a large vertical design which provides gross stimulation to fusion with most of the design common to both eyes; the D series, the Wells ON NE design, provides a third of the total design for fusion; while the E series, the HOT DOG cards, introduce some stereopsis. The M series, three wise monkeys, present a pictorial design with finer detail.

'Three cats' exercise

Many stereoscope cards or a specially designed 'cats' card may be used for this exercise. It has two line drawings of cats side by side and separated by about 5 cm from centre to centre. Usually each cat is incomplete in some way, an ear, an eye or the tail is missing, say, so that only when the two are fused is a complete cat formed. This method does not require a stereoscope.

The exercise is particularly useful for exophoric conditions when used in the following way (see *Figure 8.10*). The card is held at about 40 cm from the patient's

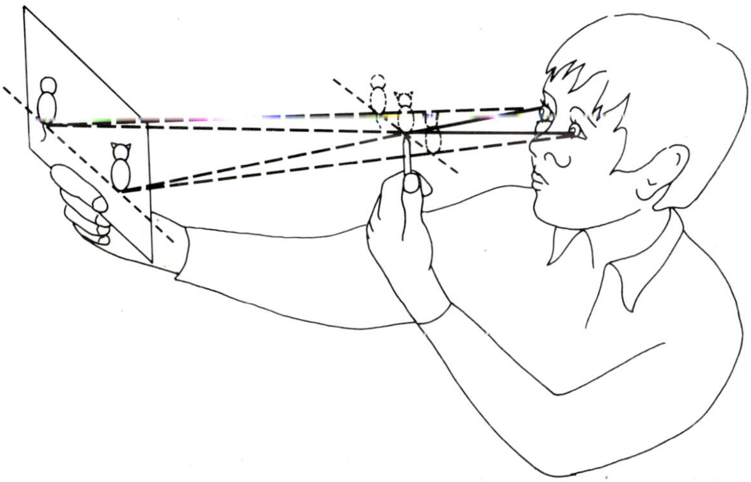

Figure 8.10. 'Three cats' exercise. The card with drawings of two incomplete cats is held at arm's length. The patient fixes a pencil held between the card and the eyes. Physiological diplopic images of the cats will be seen as blurred images, and the pencil distance adjusted until the middle two cats fuse into a complete cat with two incomplete, one each side – three cats. The patient is asked to try to see the cats clearly; to converge for the pencil distance and relax accommodation, that is, to exercise negative relative accommodation

eyes, and the patient is asked to fix the point of a pencil held mid-way between the card and the eyes. The card will then be seen in physiological diplopia – four cats instead of two. A slight adjustment of the distance of the pencil will enable the middle two cats to be fused into a complete cat with an incomplete cat on each side – the three cats. The patient is then asked to try to maintain fusion and to see the cats clearly. This requires convergence to the distance of the pencil, but exerting accommodation only for the greater distance at which the card is held. This exercises the negative relative accommodation. With practice, a clear view of the three cats can be maintained, even when the pencil has been removed. Many patients can teach themselves to exercise voluntary convergence, or 'squinting in', and obtain fusion of the cats without the use of a pencil.

This exercise can also be used for esophoric conditions, but patients tend to have more difficulties initially. It is easier if a stereoscope card is used with a small picture separation, say 3 or 4 cm; one of the early cards of the C series in the Bradford Set of Stereoscope Cards is appropriate. With esophoria, the patient is asked to fix a distant object just over the top of the card, which is held at about 30 cm before the eyes. When physiological diplopia of the two pictures on the card is appreciated, the card distance is adjusted to obtain fusion of the middle two picture designs. Fusion is maintained as the card is moved upwards slightly and thus obscures the initial fixation object. It is likely that the card will appear very blurred at first, but the patient should concentrate on maintaining fusion with under-convergence rather than clear vision at this stage. When this can be done, it is useful in obtaining clear vision if the card is moved away from the eyes to about 40 cm, where clear vision may be easier. When the fused middle picture with an incomplete one each side can be seen clearly, the patient is exercising the positive relative accommodation; that is, accommodating for the card distance while maintaining vergence appropriate to distance vision. This is not a very easy exercise to use with esophoria, and it may be more useful to keep to the use of Holmes stereoscope procedures with these patients.

When undertaking this exercise, it is very easy for exophoric patients to discover how to obtain fusion into the three cats by under-converging or for esophoric patients to fuse by over-converging. That is, patients do the exercise the wrong way round, and if this is undetected they can be exercising the wrong function.

Small hand (or Remy) diploscope

A card, at 30 cm from the eyes, contains the letters D O G. A septum, 7 cm in front of the card, has two holes in the plane of the letters which is in physiological diplopia when the eyes are looking at the card and the letters can be seen through these holes (see *Figure 8.11*). It is so arranged that the letter O is seen with both eyes, D (on the left) with the right eye only, and G (on the right) with only the left eye. The instrument provides only a very small binocular lock; the letter O. Therefore, the normal binocular position of the eyes is difficult to maintain if there is decompensated heterophoria, and in these cases the correct position of the letters, D O G, is not sustained. In esophoria, the patient may see D G or O G D O, and in exophoria D O O G. The instrument, therefore, can provide a test for decompensation. In using the instrument for exercising, the patient is encouraged to see the normal response and then go on to see the opposite appearance;

	In esophoria	*In exophoria*
Patient sees:	DG	D O O G
Patient is encouraged to see:	D O G	D O G
After exercise, patient is encouraged to see:	D O O G	DG

Coloured patches, green above and red below the letter O, can be seen through two further holes in the septum, and these assist in analysing any fixation disparity that may occur with the test.

Flip prism method

The 'flip prisms' consist of two pairs of prisms mounted on a horizontal bar, one pair (base-in) on the top of the bar and the other pair (base-out) below. One pair of prisms can be held before the eyes, and then quickly changed for the other pair by a simple flip movement made by twisting the bar extension handle. Suitable prism powers are 5^{Δ} base-in and 15^{Δ} base-out, or 4^{Δ} base-in/12^{Δ} base-out – the base-out being three times the base-in (see *Figure 8.11*).

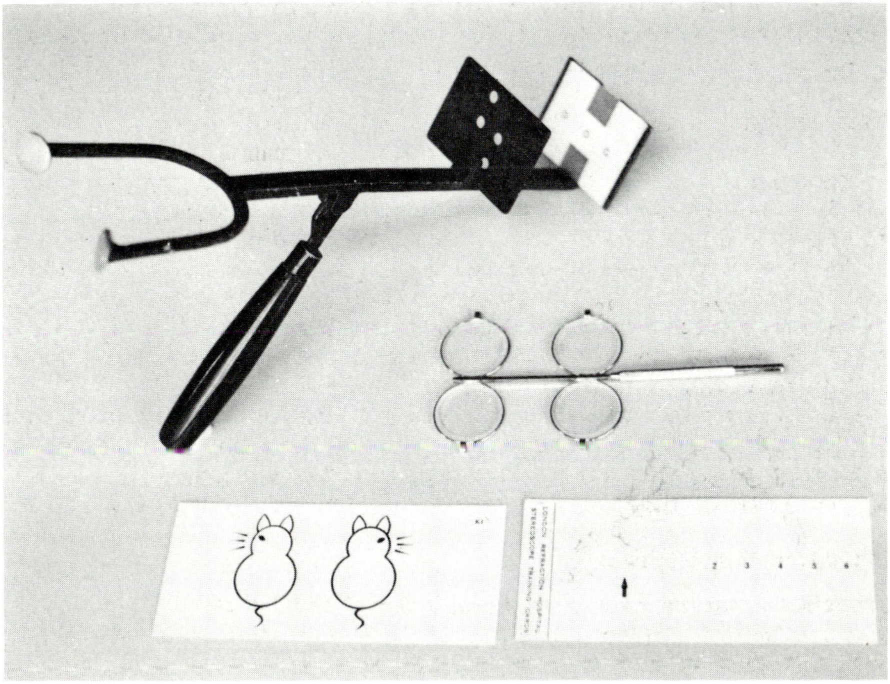

Figure 8.11. The Remy small hand diploscope (top), flip prisms (centre), 'three cats' card (left) and card for estimating picture separation in Holmes stereoscope (courtesy London Refraction Hospital)

Patients should be able to change their vergence and maintain accommodation as the prism is changed from base-in to base-out and back again. Exercising with flip prisms is carried out by asking the patient to look at a card with fairly large letters printed on it and held at about 40 cm, while the prisms are flipped from base-in to base-out and back. It should be possible to execute 20 complete cycles per minute, and maintain this over a period of several minutes. This is known as testing the 'stamina of vergence' (Griffin, 1983).

Flip lenses

As the patient should be able to respond to the flip prisms by prompt changes of convergence, changes in relative accommodation should be made promptly also. This can be tested and exercised by flip lenses of +2 DS/−2 DS. A normal young subject can make binocular changes of 10–15 complete cycles per minute, positive to negative and back. With abnormal patients, it is important to monitor any suppression while this is taking place. This can be done with the use of the near Mallett unit. As a home exerciser, it is adequate to use the lenses flipper with a normal page of print at the usual reading distance, and to check for suppression at each visit of the patient. This 'rocking' exercise should be carried out for a few minutes several times a day. Patients usually respond in one or two weeks.

Patients with accommodative problems may also benefit from this type of exercise. This may be indicated in three functional accommodative anomalies:

(1) *Accommodative insufficiency*, in which there is a low amplitude of accommodation for the patient's age, in spite of there being no uncorrected hyperopia. The exercise does not help in those cases where there is convergence insufficiency as well as the low accommodative amplitude; these patients are best helped by a small reading addition and base-in prisms (see the management of convergence insufficiency in Chapter 6).
(2) *Accommodative fatigue* is indicated when a patient reports that accommodation cannot be sustained for long periods of near vision, but reports blurring after a short time. Again, this may be a symptom of uncorrected hyperopia, and attention should be given to this before embarking on a course of exercises.
(3) *Inert accommodation*; the accommodation responds only slowly to changes of fixation, and the patient reports that when looking from near to distance vision, or the other way, objects come into focus only after a short delay. This can also be an early sign of spasm of accommodation caused by excessive amounts of work at too close a working distance, often accompanied by uncorrected hyperopia (see Convergence excess esophoria in Chapter 5).

It will be seen that in all three cases the patient needs to have a correction for any hyperopia before orthoptic treatment for accommodative insufficiency, fatigue or inert accommodation. Active pathology as a cause of the accommodative problem should also be ruled out. Patients who will respond to the flip lenses type of exercise are usually in the age range 10–25 years. The exercise can also be preceded by a 'push-up' exercise, carried out as if repeating the measurement of amplitude of accommodation.

Synoptophore

Exercises of the prism vergence type can also be carried out with a major haplopscope using 'fusion slides'. The restricted field, stimulation of proximal convergence and other disadvantages of this type of instrument do not seem to affect the building up of fusional reserves. However, this major instrument is hardly necessary for heterophoria problems.

General co-ordination and convergence exercises

In addition to the treatment for small central suppression areas, and exercises for increasing the relative convergence and accommodation, it is sometimes useful to use procedures that exercise the accommodation and convergence in their normal relationship. It seems that when heterophoria becomes decompensated, some patients experience difficulty in interpreting the cues which stimulate the right degree of vergence change. In these cases, the disparate images of an object not at the fixation distance (in physiological diplopia) are misinterpreted. A patient with convergence excess esophoria, for example, when asked to change fixation from a near object to look at one slightly further away from the eyes, will make a divergent movement only with one eye. This will leave the eyes in the position of a temporary convergent squint. Suppression and abnormal correspondence may be produced, leading to a more permanent squint (Gillie and Lindsay, 1969). This occurs mainly in young children before the binocular reflexes are firmly established, i.e. earlier than the age of 7 years. Such patients may benefit by general co-ordination exercises, which are based largely on teaching a correct interpretation of physiological diplopia.

Older patients may also benefit from procedures which exercise the accommodation and convergence in the normal relationship. These are cases in which either the convergence or the accommodation amplitudes are low, and may be improved by 'push-up' type exercises.

Physiological diplopia

The patient is taught a proper appreciation of physiological diplopia by using two objects held on the median line against a plain background (see *Figure 8.3*). The patient fixes the more distant pencil, and should see the nearer one in crossed physiological diplopia. It helps if the pencils (or knitting needles) are of a different colour. When crossed physiological diplopia has been appreciated, the patient is asked to change fixation to the nearer pencil and to notice that the other is in uncrossed diplopia. The exercise consists of fixation of one pencil, pausing long enough to be sure that it is single while the other is in physiological diplopia, and then changing fixation to establish single vision of the other with diplopia of the first. This alternation of fixation should not be carried out too fast or confusion results; there should be a 3-second pause at each change to ensure the correct interpretation has been made. At first, the patient's eyes should be observed to see the steady and regular change of vergence of both eyes.

When this can be carried out successfully using isolated objects like the two pencils or two knitting needles against a plain background, the patient can be taught to appreciate physiological diplopia at any time by holding up a pencil or a finger and noticing the doubling of objects beyond. A change of fixation to the distant object will produce diplopia of the pencil.

In the case of exophoric conditions and in convergence insufficiency, the nearer object should be held at about 40 cm from the eyes to begin with, and moved closer when this jump convergence exercise can be carried out successfully at this distance. It should be possible to perform the exercise with the nearer object at 10 cm before the treatment is finished.

The bead-on-string exercise, described earlier in the chapter, is also very useful as a home exercise, and is an extension of the physiological diplopia principle (see *Figure 8.7*).

Pencil-to-nose exercises

These exercises have been found useful in exophoric conditions in convergence insufficiency for many years. This type of exercise can be essentially a variant on the physiological diplopia exercise above. The patient is asked to look at a pencil placed at about 50 cm or well outside the range of the near point convergence. It is then moved towards the eyes until it appears double, or the practitioner sees that one eye has ceased to converge. This is repeated until the amplitude of convergence is closer than 10 cm. If diplopia is not appreciated as soon as the practitioner notices that one eye has ceased to converge, physiological diplopia of some distant object should be appreciated and the increased separation of these images observed as the pencil is brought closer to the nose.

Duration of Exercises

Usually patients should be encouraged to practise orthoptic exercises for several ten minute periods each day. In the case of young children, it may be necessary to give more than one exercise or to change the details slightly such as giving more than one set of stereoscope cards. This helps to maintain interest. Some exercises requiring little apparatus can be carried out frequently at odd moments during the day.

Patients should be seen at least once a week to check the progress and encourage persistence with the exercises. Some conditions respond more quickly, but in general exercises for one objective need to be pursued for at least several weeks. It is wise to continue for two weeks after the objective of the exercise appears to have been achieved in order to consolidate the progress made.

References

ASHER, H. and LAW, F. W. (1952). Stereoscopy: a new stereoscope. *British Journal of Ophthalmology*, **36,** 225

EARNSHAW, J. (1960). The use of knitting needles in the treatment of strabismus. *Optician*, **139,** 465–466

GILLIE, J. C. and LINDSAY, M. A. (1969). *Orthoptics*. Hatton Press, London, pp. 50–60

GRIFFIN, J. R. (1983). *Binocular Anomalies*. Professional Press, Chicago, p. 401

HUMPHRISS, D. (1953). Divergence excess, etiology and treatment. *British Journal of Physiological Optics*, **10**(1), 27–38

LYLE, T. K. and WYBAR, K. C. (1967). *Practical Orthoptics in the Treatment of Squint*. Lewis, London, p. 146

PICKWELL, L. D. (1971). Simple methods in everyday orthoptics. *Optician*, **161**(4177), 10–12

PICKWELL, L. D. (1979). Prevalence and management of divergence excess. *American Journal of Optometry*, **56**(2), 8

LTL

9

Anisometropia and aniseikonia

Binocular vision can be disturbed by large differences in the refractive error between the two eyes. This is known as 'anisometropia'. When this is left uncorrected, central retinal suppression areas can develop in the eye with the more blurred vision. If this occurs in young patients, and particularly before the age of 6 years when the visual system is still not firmly established, amblyopia may also be present. Often in these cases, the vision is very good in one eye, so that the anisometropia and reduced vision in the other is not discovered. The older the child, the more difficult it is to treat the amblyopia and restore full acuity. The importance of early eye examination is obvious, and the procedures for the examination of young children are dealt with in Chapter 15. There is no doubt that a lot of anisometropic amblyopia is preventable by early examination and correction by spectacles. The treatment of anisometropic amblyopia is covered in Chapter 11, together with other types of functional amblyopia.

With patients of any age, the prescribing of glasses to correct anisometropia may present two other problems:

(1) *Prismatic effects* – when the patient is not looking through the optical centres of the lenses, a difference in prismatic effect between the two lenses can make binocular vision difficult or impossible. These prismatic effects present more difficulties when the patient looks above or below the centres, as the vertical tolerance to prisms is very much less than the horizontal.
(2) *Aniseikonia* – when the lenses are of different powers, there will be a larger retinal image in one eye than the other due to the difference in spectacle magnification.

In both cases, these difficulties will cause more problems in older patients, with previously uncorrected patients or where a large change in prescription is given.

Prismatic effects

Diagnosis

The main factor in recognizing a difficulty due to prismatic effects in the peripheral vision of the patient when looking through the spectacles, is the presence of the anisometropia itself. It may also be found that older children and teenage patients with anisometropia have spasm of accommodation, and where this is suspected a cycloplegic refraction should be carried out. The symptoms of the anisometropia will be those due to the type of refractive error in the better eye – headache for near vision in hyperopia and blurred distance vision in myopia. Some patients may be hyperopic in one eye and myopic in the other. In these cases, they may use one eye for distance vision and the other for close work. If there is no refractive error in one eye, the patient may have no symptoms. This may also be true in cases where no glasses have been worn and suppression has developed.

Many patients will experience no problems when spectacles are prescribed; the younger the patient when glasses are first worn, the more likely that trouble can be avoided. This is probably because patients with stable binocular vision or compensated heterophoria can adapt to prism in a very short time. The symptoms that occur when the patient does not adapt to the correction for anisometropia consist of difficulties in getting used to the new glasses – headache or intermittent diplopia. Troubles seldom occur when the anisometropia is less than 2 D.

Management

Often, these difficulties can be avoided by anticipation. A partial correction is given in the more hyperopic eye in those cases where there has been no previous correction or where there is a large difference between the previous correction and the new one. The extent of this modification to the prescription can be determined by the infinity balance 'nodding test': the patient looks at the letters L and F on the infinity balance (or septum test) through the full correction, and is asked to move the head vertically up and down in a nodding movement so that the eyes look through the lenses above and then below the optical centres. If the patient reports an apparent vertical movement of the two letters relative to each other, the prescription is modified until they do not appear to move significantly during the nodding. An alternative method is to carry out the cover test with the eyes looking through the near visual points and again when looking through the optical centres. The power of the more positive lens is reduced until a good recovery movement to the induced hyperphoria occurs.

As a rough guide, the prescription for the more hyperopic eye is reduced by one-third of the change in the anisometropia (the difference between the two eyes) compared with the previous prescription. This will mean that it is reduced by one-third of the anisometropia in the case of a patient who has worn no previous glasses. However, it must not be assumed that all patients with anisometropia will experience difficulties with their new glasses. Some patients with marked anisometropia will settle very readily to a new prescription, whereas others with low degrees will experience symptoms.

Patients often learn very quickly to turn the head rather than the eyes, so that they always look through the optical centres of the lenses. It is sometimes helps to encourage patients to do this. Another very useful approach is to fit contact lenses, which move with the eyes so that no prismatic effect is induced. Contact lenses can also help with size difference in some cases.

Aniseikonia due to spectacle magnification differences

Diagnosis

Most aniseikonia arises from the difference in spectacle magnification that accompanies anisometropic corrections; this type may be called 'acquired optical aniseikonia'. Other types will be considered separately later in this chapter.

Diagnosis that aniseikonic problems are likely to occur can be foreseen largely from the presence of the anisometropia, and particularly when there is a difference in spectacle magnification of more than 1%. Again, symptoms will consist of the non-tolerance of the new glasses, and sometimes headache and intermittent diplopia. A symptom more characteristic of aniseikonia is a disturbance in spatial perception; the floor appears to slope or other horizontal objects appear tilted when looking through the new glasses. Investigation with an eikonometer may be carried out, but this is very unusual as most practitioners do not have the apparatus. Its use may be more necessary in types of aniseikonia other than acquired optical, and will therefore be considered together with them.

Management

Anticipation of the difficulties is again very important in dealing with these cases. The following should be considered:

(1) Warn the patient that difficulties in space perception may occur during the first few days of wearing the new glasses. It is usually adequate to say that the patient's particular prescription is of the type that may require a few days to

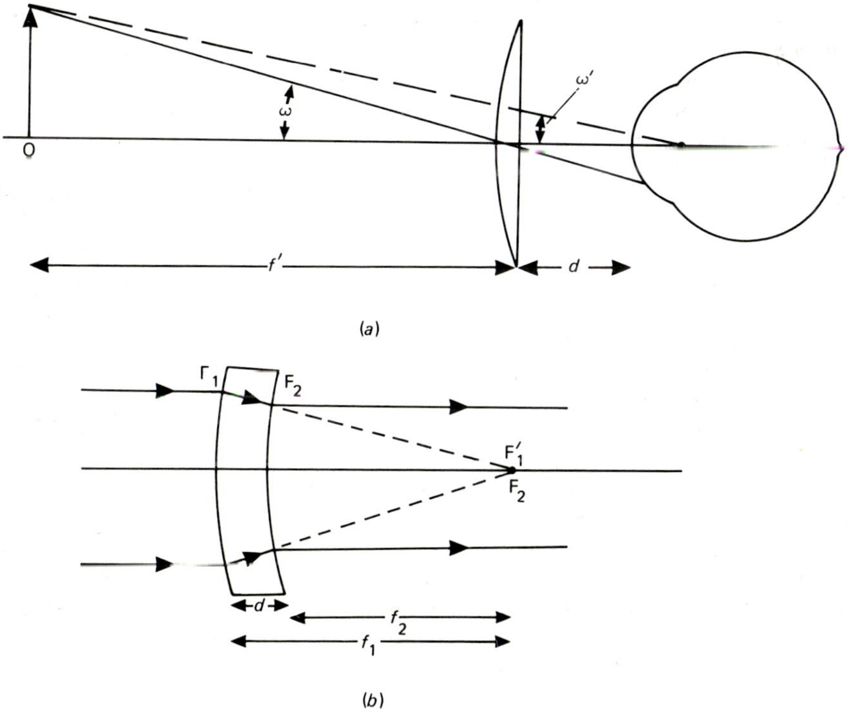

Figure 9.1. (a) The spectacle magnification (SM) is the ratio of the angle subtended at the eye by the object to the angle subtended at the spectacle lens. This can be shown to be SM = $1/(1-d \cdot F)$, where d is the spectacle distance, and F the power of the lens. As the lens is moved closer to the eye (d decreases), spectacle magnification will become unity. As the power of the lens (F) increases, the spectacle magnification will increase. (b) The magnification of a 'thick' lens is the ratio between the focal lengths of the surface powers. This can be shown to be $1/(1+t \cdot F_1)$, where F_1 is the power of the front surface, and t is the reduced thickness of the lens (d/n)

settle to the new glasses. In most cases, these problems will diasppear after a short time, particularly if some of the factors mentioned below have been considered.

(2) Reduce the difference in spectacle magnification by considering the factors that contribute to it (see *Figure 9.1*).
   (a) *Lens power* – the higher the power, the higher the spectacle magnification. A partial correction for one eye can be considered, again on the basis of reducing by about one-third of the change in the anisometropia. In some cases, a partial correction in both eyes may be appropriate, as this will leave the patient to exert the same accommodative effort in both eyes. With young patients, such a binocular reduction will give sufficient correction to relieve any symptoms of hyperopia, but because both lenses are less powerful, the difference in spectacle magnification will be less.
   (b) *Lens form* – the deeper the meniscus (i.e. the higher the base curve), the greater the spectacle magnification. The lenses should be dispensed with the more positive lens in a 'flatter' form than the other. This will reduce the spectacle magnification a little, and it will also result in the front surfaces of the lenses being more similar in appearance.
   (c) *Lens thickness* – the thicker the lens, the greater the spectacle magnification. The least powerful positive lens can be thicker than normal, so that its spectacle magnification is increased slightly. This will also have the effect of helping to balance the weight of the two lenses. Clearly, the more powerful lens needs to be kept as thin as is consistent with the type of frame or mount used. This will maintain the spectacle magnification and the weight at a minimum.
   (d) *Spectacle distance* – the closer the lens is to the eyes, the less will be the spectacle magnification. It is not possible to mount one lens closer to the eyes than the other, but if the spectacle distance is kept to a minimum, the spectacle magnification for both eyes will be at a minimum and therefore the difference between them less.

(3) Contact lenses can be considered, as these provide the greatest reduction in the spectacle distance. It has already been noted that contact lenses also help to overcome the difficulties which arise from differential prismatic effect.

Astigmatic corrections

These factors can help to reduce the difference in spectacle magnification to a degree where it is unlikely to cause problems in those cases where the anisometropia is mainly spherical. Where the anisometropia is astigmatic, requiring a higher cylindrical correction in one eye than the other, or where there are high cylinders in both eyes, it is much more likely that there will be disturbances in space perception due to the meridional magnification. The factors mentioned above will assist in these cases, too. Warn the patient of the likely disturbances during the first few days of wearing the new glasses. Consider a partial astigmatic correction, and keep the spectacle distance to a minimum.

Lens thickness and form can be employed to overcome the problems in astigmatic corrections by prescribing 'isogonal' lenses (Halass, 1959). These are lenses whose thickness and surface powers have to be calculated to produce the same spectacle magnification in both meridians of both lenses: there is no difference in spectacle magnification to create aniseikonia. Usually, isogonal lenses require to be made with a toric surface on both sides of each lens, with the principal meridans parallel on each side. This is a very difficult and an expensive process, and therefore isogonal lenses are only prescribed where other methods of relieving the symptoms of the aniseikonia have failed. It should be noted, however, that an eikonometer is not required for prescribing isogonal lenses.

Contact lenses are effective in reducing the problems with astigmatic aniseikonia, and when other factors make the patient appropriate for contact lens wear, this is the most satisfactory method.

Other types of aniseikonia

It is also possible that aniseikonia can be the result of differences that are inherent in the visual system; a difference in the optical system or length of the eyes, or due to an anomaly in the arrangement of the neurons of the two eyes – 'anatomical aniseikonia'. These differences are likely to be present at birth, from an early age or to come on very gradually. In many cases, the visual system adapts to the difference, and either tolerates it or suppresses one eye. Where suppression occurs, no method of detecting the aniseikonia is available, unless the suppression is treated.

Where the aniseikonia is of a degree to be tolerated, it is possible that some change can result in it becoming intolerable and symptoms occur. Diagnosis in these cases requires an eikonometer. There are two types of eikonometer:

(1) *Ames eikonometer*, which presents a separate image to each eye so that the patient can make a direct comparison of the image sizes.
(2) *Space eikonometer*, which allows the patient to recognize distortions of space perception, such as a tilting of the frontoparallel plane out of its normally perceived position.

In both cases, measurement of image size differences are made by incorporating an afocal optical system of variable magnification which is adjusted until a normal appearance is reported by the patient. Neither of these instruments gives very consistent results. A number of readings is taken, and if the spread of readings is less than the mean value, this mean value may be taken as the size difference. A 'size-lens' (or aniseikonic lens) can be prescribed to give this magnification. As with isogonal lenses, the thickness and surface curves are calculated to give the required magnification. Again, if there is an astigmatic element or if a meridional magnification is required, a size-lens will require two toric surfaces.

Because of the cost of making a size-lens to a patient's individual prescription, and also because of the indefinite nature of eikonometer readings, trial periods of wearing afocal size-lenses are sometimes undertaken. A stock size-lens of approximately the magnification required is worn for several days clipped on the patient's normal glasses. It is tried so that it equalizes the image sizes, and also for a few days before the other eye so that it increases the size difference. In the first case it should alleviate the symptoms, and in the second make them temporarily worse. This will verify that it is the aniseikonia which is causing the problems and that a size-lens would be appropriate to alleviate them.

Reference

HALASS, S. (1959). Aniseikonic lenses of improved design and their application. *Australian Journal of Optometry*, **42**, 387–393

Part III

Squint

10

Sensory changes in squint

Diplopia and confusion

If a squint occurs before the patient reaches the age of about 3 years, binocular vision will not have become firmly established, so that the visual system may adapt to the deviation without the patient experiencing symptoms. On the other hand, when a squint is acquired by an adult, symptoms are very likely to occur because retinal correspondence has become established between the two eyes and predominantly between the central foveal areas. In such cases, the correspondence between the two eyes may embarrass the binocular vision in two ways:

(1) *Diplopia* – the image of the object that the patient is looking at will fall on the fovea of the dominant eye and on a peripheral area of the deviated eye (see *Figure 10.1*). Normal correspondence will result in the object being located in two visual directions: the patient may describe these as one being straight ahead and the other in the periphery of vision. That is, the patient will experience diplopia as the retinal images do not fall on normally corresponding points.

(2) *Confusion* – the fovea of the deviating eye will also receive an image of some object other than that of the patient's attention. Because of the correspondence between the two eyes, the central image of the fixing eye will be confused by the cortical superimposition of the different central image in the deviated eye. When the two predominantly corresponding areas receive different images, a state of 'retinal rivalry' is present and it is likely that one image will be suppressed from consciousness over a small central area. A changing pattern of retinal rivalry will occur over the rest of the visual field. Stimulation of normally corresponding points by different images presents the situation which is known as confusion.

In young patients, adaptations to the visual system are likely, so that diplopia and confusion are not experienced by the patient. These adaptations consist of:

(a) an adaption of the localization mechanism, or the *'where system'*, which is probably mediated by the *'y'* cells from the peripheral areas of the retina; and/or

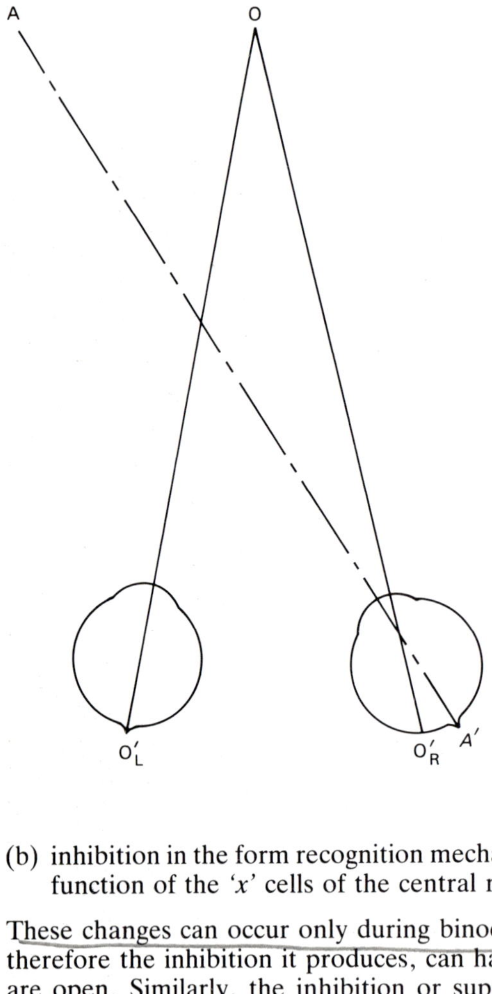

Figure 10.1. Binocular vision in right convergent squint: when the patient looks at some object O, the image of this object will fall on the fovea of the undeviated left eye, at O'_L. In the deviated right eye, the image of the object will fall on some other retinal area nasal to the fovea, at O'_R, As these two points, O'_L and O'_R, are not normally corresponding points, the object will be given two visual directions by the visual system, i.e. it will be seen in diplopia. As O'_R falls on the nasal retina in the right eye, it will be seen to the right of the left eye image – in uncrossed diplopia. The fovea of the deviated eye will receive the image of some other object, A. As there is normally a correspondence between the right fovea and the left fovea, confusion can occur between these two different images, A′ and O'_L, which will lead to retinal rivalry and eventually to suppression in young patients

(b) inhibition in the form recognition mechanism, or the '*what system*', which is the function of the '*x*' cells of the central retina.

These changes can occur only during binocular vision. This type of diplopia, and therefore the inhibition it produces, can have no meaning except when both eyes are open. Similarly, the inhibition or suppression of the central image and any abnormal extension of the Panum's fusional areas is evoked by the binocular confusion. Adaptations to the 'where system' are traditionally known as 'abnormal retinal correspondence' (ARC), and are present in the retinal area which receives the peripheral image of the object of regard in the squinting eye, so that the location of images in this area cannot be determined correctly. The condition in which there is inhibition of the 'what system' in the central area of the retina is known clinically as 'suppression' (see *Figure 10.2*).

There are two other sensory changes that may be present in squint, and these are monocular. They occur in the squinting eye of a unilateral squint, and remain when the other eye is covered. Indeed, the dominant eye needs to be covered to detect and investigate them. They are amblyopia and eccentric fixation.

These sensory changes which occur in squint developing at an early age are more fully described in the following two chapters, which deal mainly with the clinical investigation and treatment of the anomalies. Before proceeding to these chapters, it is useful to summarize something more of the nature of both the monocular and the binocular changes.

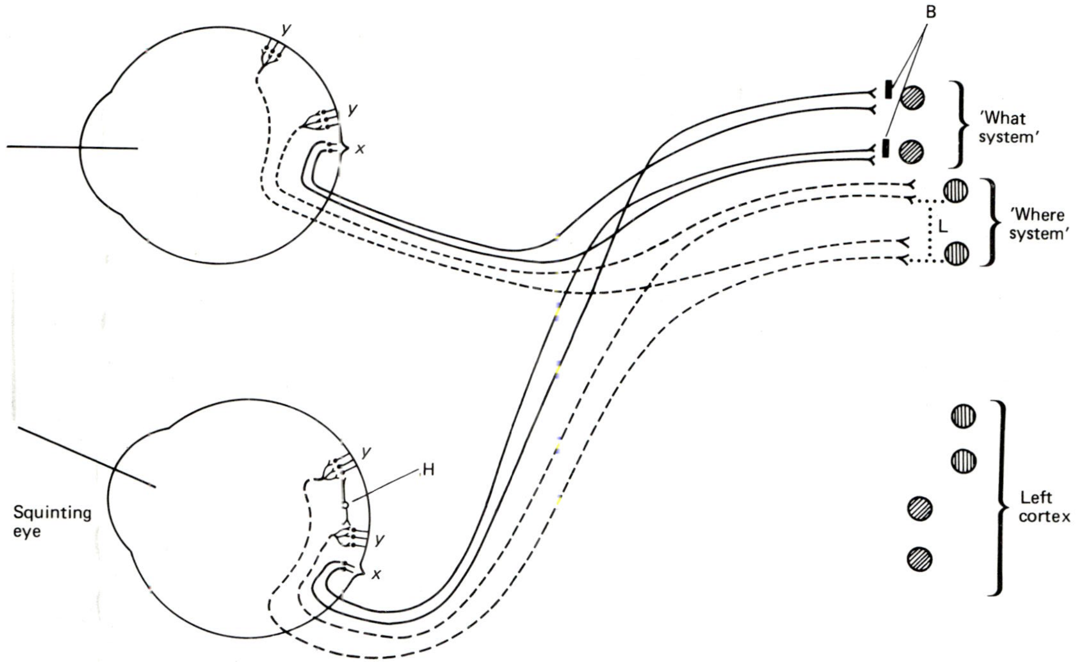

Figure 10.2. Sensory adaptations in squint – possible mechanism. Each eye has two systems: the 'what system' and the 'where system'. The first of these is responsible for form vision and is medicated by the '*x*-cell' pathway from the central retinal area. The 'where system' provides information about the position of objects, so that accurate fixation movements can be made. It is mediated by the '*y*-cell' pathway from the peripheral retina to a different part of the brain's cortex. When the cortical cells responsible for form vision receive different neural images from the two eyes, that from the non-dominant squinting eye is inhibited or blocked, possibly at B, giving rise to the clinical entity known as suppression. The 'where system' may be adapted in squint when normally corresponding points receive different images. A loss of resolution in the system occurs because retinal units over an abnormally large area are connected to each other instead of transmitting separate neural signals; there is convergence of nerve paths. This could occur at several levels in the nerve path; for example, either at the level of the retinal horizontal cells, H, or in the brain at L. It could also be at the level of the lateral geniculate bodies which are not shown in the figure, which is intended to illustrate the principle of the adaptation and is not a precise anatomical diagram

Monocular changes

Amblyopia

This is a reduction of form vision with no obvious organic cause. In squint cases, it may assist in lessening the effects of confusion, but there are other types of amblyopia which do not necessarily accompany squint. These also will be discussed in Chapter 11. Amblyopia may be partial and show as a reduction of the acuity, or in extreme cases there may be a small central scotoma.

Eccentric fixation

This is a failure of an eye in monocular vision to take up fixation with the fovea. It is thought to occur when the central acuity has dropped to a level below that of the area round the fovea, so that slight eccentric fixation gives better acuity when the other eye is covered (Worth, 1906). There has also been a suggestion that it arises from a change of the central area of localization as a central scotoma develops in the amblyopic eye (Duke-Elder, 1973). It has also been suggested that eccentric fixation occurs in squint because of a failure of the extrinsic ocular muscle to relax from the deviation – muscle potentiation (Schor, 1978). In other patients, it may be a sequel to an enlargement of Panum's fusion area which follows decompensated heterophoria at an early age and leads eventually to microsquint (Pickwell, 1981).

These different reasons for eccentric fixation are not necessarily mutually exclusive. One or more may apply to a particular patient, and the others in other patients. Usually, there are no accompanying changes to the localization system in the monocular vision of an eccentrically fixing eye. The image on the eccentric retinal area which is used for fixation continues to be localized eccentrically; that is, the visual direction normally associated with the eccentric area still applies. Patients describe the object of regard during monocular vision as appearing to be slightly to one side, and not straight ahead. This type of anomaly, eccentric fixation without the loss of normal centralization, is sometimes referred to as 'eccentric viewing'.

The loss of central localization in eccentric fixation cases during monocular vision may occur, but usually the acuity is so poor that the condition is very difficult to investigate.

Binocular changes

Suppression

This is an inhibition of images from a central area of the retina of one eye during binocular conditions. It may be thought of as a suppression scotoma in the squinting eye when, due to the deviation, the corresponding retinal area of the other eye is receiving a different image. If the undeviated eye is covered, the squinting eye will take up fixation, either centrally or eccentrically, and the suppression scotoma will no longer be present. It is an inhibition of form vision, and as such it will be present predominantly in the central region of the retina. In convergent squint, the suppression area may extend into the nasal retina so as to cover the retina area which normally receives the image of the object of regard. In divergent squint, it may extend into the temporal retina or may even include most of the retina of the squinting eye – total suppression.

Abnormal retinal correspondence

This is an adaptation of an area of the retina in the squinting eye so that all the receptors responsible for visual direction have the same 'local sign'; they localize any image falling on the area in the same direction as a single retinal point, or normal size Panum's area, in the other eye. This occurs only during binocular vision. If the non-squinting eye is covered, the squinting eye takes up fixation, and each of the receptors assumes its normal local sign or visual direction. In binocular vision, the squinting eye has an extended area which acts like an enlarged Panum's area and corresponds with a single retinal point in the other eye – a 'pseudo-Panum's area' (Bagolini, 1972). Where this pseudo-Panum's area corresponds with the fovea of the other eye, the condition is known as 'harmonious abnormal retinal correspondence'. This is the case in over 90% of squints. In other cases, the pseudo-Panum's area appears to be centred nearer the fovea of the

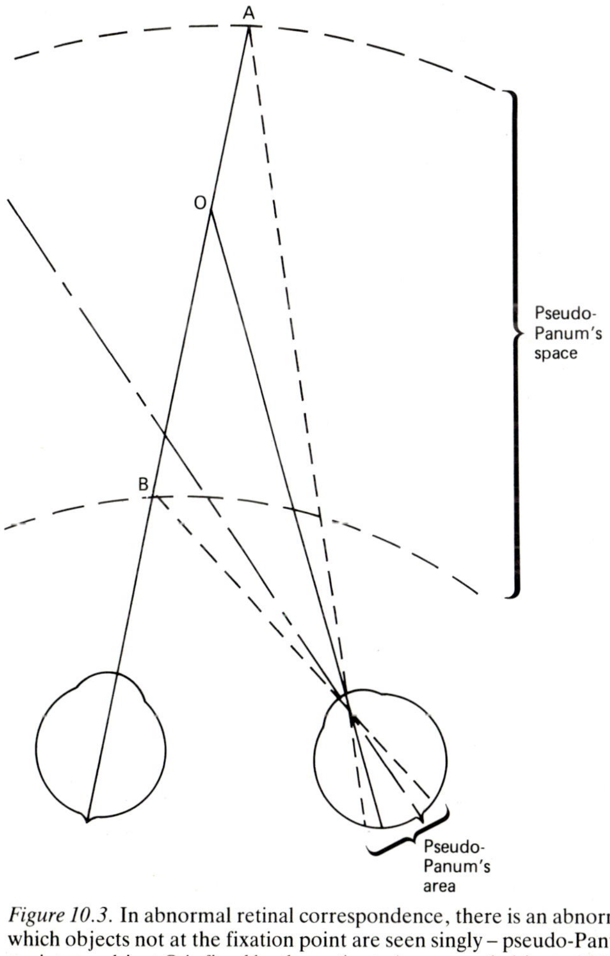

Figure 10.3. In abnormal retinal correspondence, there is an abnormal extension of the spatial area in which objects not at the fixation point are seen singly – pseudo-Panum's space. In right convergent squint, an object O is fixed by the patient. Any second object within pseudo-Panum's space, between A and B, will not appear to be double. This is a much larger area than Panum's space in normal subjects, and extends to include the macular field in most squinting patients. Similarly, there is a pseudo-Panum's area of the retina which is larger than in normal subjects

squinting eye and is called 'inharmonious' or 'incongruous' abnormal retinal correspondence. It may be the result of the angle of the squint having been changed by operation.

As images falling on the pseudo-Panum's area of the squinting eye correspond with the fovea in most patients, they will have the same visual direction (see *Figure 10.3*). Therefore, the object of regard by the squinting patient has the same visual direction for both eyes in spite of the squint, and there will be no diplopia. Put in another way, abnormal retinal correspondence is an adaptation to the localization system, which avoids diplopia by giving the images in both eyes the same visual direction in spite of the squint.

In most patients who have a squint from an early age, both suppression and abnormal retinal correspondence are present. In convergent squint, form vision is suppressed in the squinting eye at the macula and into the nasal retina to the point which receives the image of the object of regard. Localization of objects in space is modified across a more extensive peripheral area of the squinting eye, so that this abnormal correspondence gives objects the same visual direction and avoids diplopia. This can be demonstrated by the use of the striate lens (see Chapter 12). The streak seen with the deviated eye usually has the central part missing, showing the suppression, and is also seen in line with the fixation light, indicating that there is abnormal correspondence. In larger angles of squint (over 15°), the streak is not seen at all with the squinting eye, indicating that all the retinal elements on the nasal retina are suppressed.

It may also be noted that there are two modifications which are known to occur normally in the nervous system. These are inhibition of a neuron, and convergence of nerve paths. In the first case, it appears that the nervous system is able to inhibit the passage of the signal through a particular junction of nerve cells and fibres, and that this is used as part of the mechanism for processing the signals. Convergence of several nerve paths to channel more than one signal into a single nerve path is also a normal part of the nervous system. These can be demonstrated in the retina where the 'horizontal' and the 'amacrine' cells perform this function, and there is some evidence that the amount of convergence of nerve paths increases as part of the mechanism of dark adaptation of the eye (Pickwell, 1980). The sensory adaptations in squint are abnormal protractions of these two mechanisms. Both suppression and abnormal retinal correspondence may be considered as abnormal uses of normal mechanisms which serve binocular interaction in normal binocular vision. They are adaptations of methods of neural functioning to compensate for the squint.

References

BAGOLINI, B. (1972). Anomalous binocular vision in strabismic patients. *2nd International Orthoptic Congress of the British Optical Association*, pp. 298–308

DUKE-ELDER, SIR STEWART (1973). *System of Ophthalmology*, vol. VI, *Ocular Motility and Strabismus*. Kimpton, London, p. 326

PICKWELL, L. D. (1980). A model for sensory adaptations of the visual system in squint. *British Journal of Ophthalmology*, **64**(5), 345–348

PICKWELL, L. D. (1981). A suggestion for the origin of eccentric fixation. *Ophthalmic and Physiological Optics*, **1**, 55–57

SCHOR, C. (1978). A motor theory for monocular eccentric fixation of amblyopic eyes. *American Journal of Optometry*, **55**, 183–186

WORTH, C. (1906). Quoted in Duke-Elder, Sir Stewart (see above), pp. 325–326

11

Amblyopia and eccentric fixation

Amblyopia

As indicated in the previous chapter, amblyopia is a loss of visual acuity of an eye with no obvious organic cause. It may show as a reduction in the patient's ability to read the smaller letters on a Snellen or other chart, or as a very small central scotoma in which there is no central vision. It is a loss in spacial frequency resolution. The term 'organic amblyopia' is also used to indicate a similar loss of acuity or central vision which can be attributed to some pathological change. This may be due to an abnormality in the visual pathway or sensory system which may have no obvious signs. It may be an innate structural defect or an acquired anomaly, as in the case of toxic amblyopia or glaucoma. It is obviously very important to each patient that any organic cause be detected, so that appropriate medical treatment can be considered. Amblyopia which is not caused by active disease processes is called 'functional amblyopia', and it is with this type that this chapter is principally concerned. Differential diagnosis between organic and functional amblyopia will also be discussed.

The main cause of functional amblyopia is deprivation of some kind and hence the term sometimes used is 'deprivation amblyopia'. Normal visual acuity in humans does not reach full development until the age of about 5 years. For full acuity to develop at all, a clear central image is required during the developmental years up to about 3. Up to the age of 5 or 6 years, the visual system is not firmly established and can readily be disturbed. If an eye is deprived of a central or a clear image before this age, development of the acuity will be arrested and amblyopia will result. Untreated unilateral squint will mean that one eye is deprived of a central image, and anisometropia or high astigmatism will present a blurred image in one or both eyes. Where this occurs before the age of 5 years, there will be deprivation amblyopia (von Noorden, 1974). It has been shown that good acuity (6/6 or 20/20) in terms of neural and optical resolution measured by electrophysiological or by optokinetic methods may be present under the age of one year. However, cognitive form recognition does not develop until about 3 years. Therefore Snellen type tests do not show good acuity until 3 years.

This emphasizes the need for early detection of the causes of amblyopia; squint and refractive error. Preventative measures and treatment can then be instituted.

An eye that is deprived of vision at an early age by being covered for a protracted period will also fail to develop acuity, due to its disuse or deprivation. This is sometimes called 'amblyopia ex anopsia', a term best reserved for these rather unusual circumstances of prolonged occlusion – lid closure, congenital cataract or corneal leucoma.

Functional amblyopia is also classified according to its likely causes as follows:

(1) *Strabismic amblyopia* – the amblyopia which accompanies a squint. This may be an adaptation to the squint (Lyle and Wybar, 1967), and brought about by the fovea of the squinting eye being deprived of a central image.
(2) *Refractive amblyopia* – a term used to describe amblyopia which seems to have refractive error as part or all of its cause:
   (a) *Anisometropic amblyopia*, in which the image in one eye is so blurred, due to the difference in refractive error between the two eyes, that it is incompatible with the other image. It will also be recalled that the fovea needs a clear image in the infant in order that full acuity will develop.
   (b) *Astigmatic amblyopia*; in high astigmatism also, amblyopia can be the result of blurred retinal images. This may be bilateral if there is uncorrected astigmatism in both eyes during the developmental period.
   (c) *Hyperopia;* high degrees of hyperopia can also cause bilateral amblyopia.

When a patient comes with reduced vision as a part of the symptoms, a full routine examination should be carried out. This is outlined in Chapter 2. The present chapter will deal with the particular procedures in the investigation of amblyopia as a part of that routine, and with supplementary tests that may be needed to reach a diagnosis with respect to the amblyopia. As a part of this investigation, tests for the presence of eccentric fixation may also be required, and these are given in a later section of this chapter.

HISTORY AND SYMPTOMS

From what has been said above, it will be clear that the age of onset of the amblyopia is very important in assessing each case, and taken together with the patient's present age it will be important in considering the likely prognosis. In the case of strabismic amblyopia, the age at which the squint was first noticed should be known. Sometimes, photographs taken a few years previously will help in assessing whether the squint was present at the time. The longer the squint has been present, the less likely it is to respond to treatment.

It is important to have a full appreciation of any previous treatment in the form of glasses, occlusion or other therapy: when was this given, what was its effect, and why was it discontinued? In the case of spectacles, the prescription should be known and the extent to which they have been worn.

ACUITY MEASUREMENT

Assessment of the unaided vision should be made, but an evaluation of amblyopia can only be made with the optimum spectacle correction in place. Acuity will vary a little with the illumination, the contrast and the type of test used, and every effort should be made to standardize the apparatus and the procedure used. This may need to vary to some extent with the age of the patient, as young children require a different approach. The method used should then be recorded along with the acuity measurement.

LTC

Line acuity
This is the most usual method. It is sometimes called 'morphoscopic acuity', and is recorded by the patient reading the smallest line from a standard chart of letters, Landolt Cs, or illiterate Es, etc. In recording acuity for patients with one amblyopic eye, it often happens that patients give up reading when the letters are too small to read easily. If pressed, however, patients can read lower down the chart, and sometimes this can be several lines better than where the patient would have given up. It is important to ask the patient to read until the real limit of acuity is reached, otherwise no real starting point for any treatment is known and any improvement may be more apparent than real. Patients may make more effort to read the chart after treatment or the practitioner may press them a little more.

The acuity of the amblyopic eye should be taken before the other eye, so that there is no question of the patient remembering letters. This is particularly important with children, but all patients find it difficult to know if a letter can actually be seen if they know what it is.

Where there is eccentric fixation, the small foveal scotoma may result in patients missing out letters or reading the line backwards more easily than in the normal way from left to right. This may be particularly true of left convergent squint (see *Figure 11.1*).

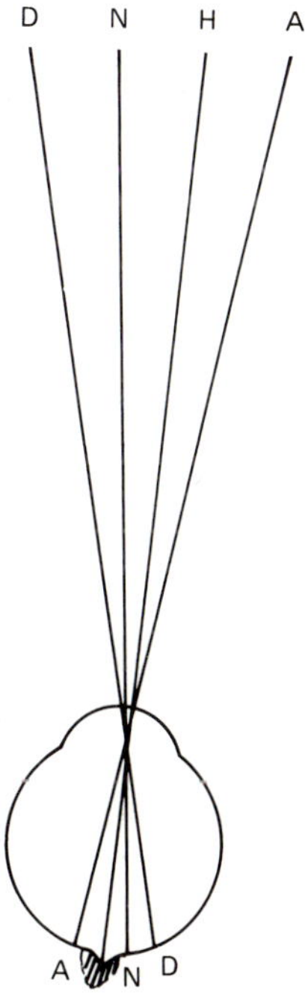

Figure 11.1. Reading Snellen letters with an eccentrically fixing eye: the patient is fixing the letter N in a line of Snellen letters. The image of the next letter on the right of N, which is H, will fall on the foveal scotoma and not be seen easily by the patient, who may therefore miss it and read the following letter, A. If the patient is asked to read from right to left instead of beginning at the left as normal, the difficulty does not occur; the image of the letter D, for example, does not fall on the scotoma

Single letter acuity
Sometimes, single letters or other characters are used instead of a line of letters, as with the E-cube or the Sheridan–Gardner test. This is also known as 'angular acuity', and is particularly useful for very young children as there is less confusion (see Chapter 15). If this method is used, there is sometimes higher acuity with

amblyopic eyes than if line acuity is measured. The term 'crowding phenomenon' is used to describe the lower acuity using a line of letters rather that single ones on a plain background. The apparant increase with single letters is called the 'separation phenomenon'. When single letter acuity is measured, the fact should be recorded with the acuity.

Neutral density filters
Re-measuring the acuity through a neutral density filter can assist in differentiating between functional amblyopia and organic amblyopia due to macular lesions, glaucoma or other organic conditions, and toxic amblyopia. A neutral density filter, ND 2, or a very dark Crookes B2 lens, is used. In eyes with normal acuity, the dark adaptation produced reduces the acuity by about a line of Snellen letters, and a similar effect occurs in anisometropic amblyopia where fixation is likely to be central. In strabismic amblyopia, however, there is usually eccentric fixation, and the amblyopic eye's acuity is not affected by the filter, as the slightly peripheral retina adapts better having a mixture of rod and cones. In organic amblyopia, there is likely to be a reduction of several lines.

Eccentric fixation

Eccentric fixation is a monocular condition in which fixation is with a point on the retina other than the fovea. Most, if not all, strabismic amblyopes have eccentric fixation. In those cases where treatment is being considered, it is important to know the degree of the eccentricity.

Tests for eccentric fixation

No method of assessing the fixation seems to be satisfactory for all patients. It is therefore important to have a number of methods available and to use those that seem most appropriate to the particular patients. It is wise to use at least two methods on each patient, and the following are suggested.

CORNEAL REFLEX TEST

Assuming that the angle lambda is the same in both eyes, a guide to eccentric fixation can be obtained by comparing the position of the corneal reflection of a pentorch in the amblyopic eye with that of the sound eye. The eye not being observed is occluded. A relative displacement of the reflex by 1 mm would indicate eccentric fixation of 11° (or 20^{Δ}), approximately. This is a large degree of eccentric fixation, but with careful observation, much smaller angles can be detected (see also Chapter 2).

PAST POINTING TEST

This will give an indication if the localization of objects in space has been disturbed with the amblyopic eye. The procedure is first tried with the patient's good eye, so that the practitioner can see the normal ability of the patient to perform the test. This is particularly useful with very young patients, and also gives such children an idea of what is expected of them. The amblyopic eye is covered, and the patient is asked to place a finger on the forehead just above the uncovered eye. A pentorch is held before the eye at a distance of about 25 cm. The practitioner explains that on the word 'Go' the patient moves the finger to touch the light. The patient is allowed to practise with the good eye if there is any difficulty. The occluder is then changed to the good eye and the test is repeated with the amblyopic eye, the patient being required to touch the light with the tip of the finger. If this cannot be done, but the finger goes a few centimetres to one side, past pointing is demonstrated. This indicates incorrect localization of the fixation point, and that the fixation does not coincide with the centre for localization.

OPHTHALMOSCOPIC METHODS

Investigation of fixation can be carried out with an ophthalmoscope which will project a target on the retina so that it can be seen by the practitioner and its position judged in relation to retinal details. As the target is focused on the retina, it can be seen by the patient and, when the patient is asked to look straight at the centre of the target, it will be seen by the practitioner to be centred on the fovea in a non-amblyopic eye. It may also be central in an amblyopic eye if the fixation is central. If it appears on any other part of the retina, usually slightly nasally in convergent squint, eccentric fixation is obviously demonstrated. Its position is recorded by a diagram.

A dilated pupil may be necessary for this type of examination, as the ophthalmoscope light is directed to the foveal area, causing pupil contraction. Also, young patients usually accommodate about 4 D when asked to look at the target from the instrument, which is very close to the eyes, and this blurs the practitioner's view of the fundus. The test is therefore better carried out during the cycloplegic refraction, when the large pupil will also increase the field of view for the practitioner and enable better location of the target on the fundus. Accommodation is also very reduced.

The eccentricity of fixation is very roughly related to the reduction in acuity (see *Figure 11.2,* which shows the acuity across the retina for a normal eye). In amblyopia, the acuity will usually be reduced a little, even for the eccentric area. As a very rough guide, the acuity will be reduced by about one line of Snellen letters for each half-degree of eccentricity of fixation. If there is anisometropia as well as a squint, there may be a further reduction in acuity.

Sometimes it is possible to place the target on the fovea, and to ask the patient what can be seen of it with the eccentrically fixing eye. Some patients report that nothing can be seen of the middle of the target, which indicates a central scotoma. Occasionally, the patients are able to give an indication of the visual direction associated with the fovea; that is, whether there is still central localization or not. The difficulty with this aspect of the investigation is maintaining the amblyopic eye's position when the target is moved from the eccentric area to the fovea. Fixation with the other eye looking at an object in a small mirror attached to a headband sometimes assists, but it is doubtful whether the information obtained by this procedure is worth the trouble.

BJERRUM SCREEN METHOD

This method depends on the fact that the physiological blind-spot is the same angular distance from the fixation point in both eyes in normal subjects.

The position of the blind-spot is plotted in the non-amblyopic eye, and the position of its centre from the fixation point horizontally and below the horizontal

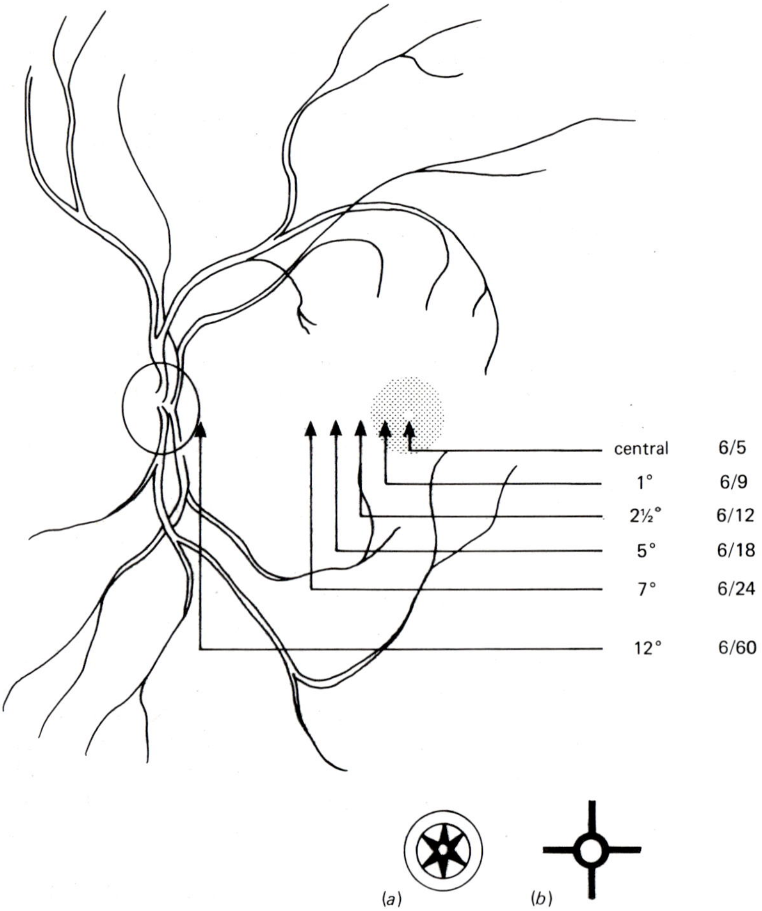

Figure 11.2. Normal variation in acuity across the retina: if the acuity of a normal eye is 6/5, the table shows an approximate acuity across the retina between the fovea and the nerve head. In amblyopes with eccentric fixation, the acuity will be lower than these values at corresponding points of fixation. (a) and (b), Examples of targets used in ophthalmoscopes for the detection of eccentric fixation

are both carefully measured. The patient is then asked to take up fixation with the amblyopic eye, the sound eye being occluded. The blind-spot is plotted for this eye and the position of the fixation spot from this is carefully compared with the sound eye. Any discrepancy between the two eyes indicates eccentric fixation (Brockbank and Downey, 1959). The position of the projection on the screen of the fovea can sometimes be estimated. A small target in this area may demonstrate a scotoma.

The co-operation from children in this method varies considerably, but it is sometimes possible to demonstrate even relatively small degrees of eccentric fixation with quite young children.

AMSLER CHARTS

These consist of 5 mm squares printed in white or in red on a black card 10 cm square. A small fixation spot is provided in the centre. A patient with a foveal scotoma will report an interruption in the pattern of the squares corresponding to the scotoma. In amblyopia with central fixation, this disturbance in the lines will be at the point of fixation and extend for about 1 cm or more, depending on the extent of the amblyopia. In eccentric fixation, the scotoma will be to one side of the point fixed by the patient – the projection of the fovea. It can extend several centimetres into the field.

The Amsler charts are also used to show early signs of organic amblyopia; for example, macular degenerations or toxic amblyopia.

AFTER-IMAGE TRANSFER METHOD

This test assumes that an after-image in one eye will be transferred to the normally corresponding point in the other; that is, a foveal after-image in the non-amblyopic eye is 'transferred' or seen with the other eye centrally.

For this test, a photographic flashgun, which has been masked to provide a very bright strip of light, is used. The amblyopic eye is occluded and the patient is asked to fix the centre of the strip with the non-amblyopic eye. The flash produces a central line after-image. The occluder is then changed to the other eye, and the patient is asked to look at a small fixation target such as a Snellen letter with the amblyopic eye. After a few seconds, the after-image appears, having been transferred at a cortical level to the amblyopic eye. The patient is asked to indicate the position of the after-image in relation to the fixation point. In eccentric fixation, the after-image will appear slightly to the side of the fixation letter.

In some cases, it can be seen a long way away – at an angular distance approaching the degree of the angle of the squint. This indicates abnormal retinal correspondence. It is comparatively unusual for there to be abnormal correspondence for after-images, and if it does occur with the after-image transfer test, it can often be overcome readily by encouraging the patient to see the after-image close to the fixation letter or passing through it. It should be noticed that the procedure in the after-image transfer method is not that normally used for the investigation of abnormal correspondence when a foveal after-image is created in both eyes and their relative spatial locations are compared.

HAIDINGER'S BRUSHES (OR MAXWELL'S SPOT) METHOD

Haidinger's brushes and Maxwell's spot are entoptic phenomena which occur due to the characteristics of the central foveal area of the retina. They can be seen only by the foveal area under the right conditions. In the case of Haidinger's brushes, a brightly illuminated blue polarized field is used. When the direction of polarization is rotated, two darkened and opposing sectors of the central field can be seen to rotate. These circumstances are created by the use of specially designed apparatus which comprises a disc of polaroid material rotating with a blue filter before a bright field – the co-ordinator. Similar apparatus can be used in some synoptophores. Maxwell's spot is seen in blue or violet light as a dark central spot. As both these phenomena are centred on the fovea, an eccentrically fixing patient will not see them at the point of fixation. If they are seen at all by such a patient, it will be slightly to the side of a fixation target. Some amblyopes cannot see the figures at all. This is particularly true where the acuity is poor – below 6/30 (Flom and Weymouth, 1961).

Evaluation, prognosis and management

When the investigation has been carried out, the practitioner will need to assess the position and decide how to proceed. Is it wise to attempt to improve the acuity, or would this risk producing intractable diplopia? It should be remembered that in some cases the amblyopia can be a consequence of a squint and helps in alleviating the diplopia and confusion. To treat the amblyopia may be a step towards treating the squint, but if it is unlikely that binocular vision can be restored, it may be better not to begin any sensory treatment. If it is decided to give treatment, it will be necessary to decide the best line to follow. Consideration should be given to the following factors:

(1) *Type of amblyopia*. Where the amblyopia appears to be the consequence of uncorrected refractive error, it is clear that the first priority will be the spectacle correction. In strabismic amblyopia, improvement of the acuity is only likely to be maintained if the treatment of the amblyopia is consolidated by the elimination of the squint – by glasses in an accommodative deviation, or by orthoptic exercises or operation in other cases. If the amblyopia is treated but the squint remains, either the amblyopia will return or diplopia will ensue.
(2) *Age of the patient*. The older the patient when treatment begins, the less likely the treatment is to be successful. Amblyopia is best treated before the age of 7 years when the vision system is still not firmly established. Some patients will respond to amblyopia treatment at a much older age, but other factors have to be favourable. Where there is eccentric fixation, it is very unlikely that central fixation will be restored in patients over the age of 5 years. The case management in such patients should aim at the best acuity, in spite of the eccentric fixation. This will not be better than the acuity associated with the area of the retina used for fixation (see *Figure 11.2*). However, this may be adequate to establish a low grade of binocular vision, perhaps a microsquint (see Chapter 13). This will give the patient some of the advantages of binocular vision, and the eyes may look straight. With large eccentricity, it is unlikely that this will occur; in microtropia, fixation is usually less that 3½° (6^Δ) eccentric. In cases of very young patients, the type of treatment may have to be determined by the patient's ability to co-operate. It may have to be confined to spectacles and occlusion, or sometimes just occlusion.
(3) *Duration of the amblyopia*. From what has been said earlier, it will be clear that the length of time that the amblyopia has been present is critical. The shorter the time since the onset of the factors causing the amblyopia, the more likely it is that the acuity can be restored. A short period of occlusion in a patient under 6 years old, with a relatively recent onset, may be very rewarding, but in a very long-standing case it would be unlikely to produce a significant improvement.
(4) *Acuity*. Some types of treatment are more appropriate where the acuity has only deteriorated to 6/24. Lower acuities usually require long periods of occlusion. Acuities worse than 6/36 in patients over the age of 6 years are unlikely to respond to treatment.
(5) *Co-operation and interest*. Active exercises are only appropriate if the patient and the parent's interest can be held. In other cases, greater reliance has to be placed on the spectacle correction or on occlusion. In the cases where occlusion is being considered, it is more likely to be effectively maintained in younger children where the patient is interested and co-operative. On the whole, younger children can be relied on to wear an occluder (patch). This is usually

not true after the early teens. Teenage patients may co-operate more with other forms of treatment if these are appropriate (Pickwell and Jenkins, 1982). Teenage patients do not like wearing an occluder and it is more difficult to persuade them to do so. On the other hand, the physiological diplopia methods seem more acceptable and it is easier for these to be understood and applied by teenagers. They require a starting acuity of better than 6/24, but it is unlikely that anything will be more successful in these older patients if the starting acuity is worse. An ability to understand what is required by the patient and the parent is important in all patients if co-operation is to be given.

CHOICE OF METHOD

Although a number of methods are available, no one method is likely to be appropriate for every patient, and some patients may require more than one type of therapy at some stage in the total management. The factors outlined above should be considered in each case. Sometimes it will be obvious where to start, and the prognosis looks good. In other cases, it is less obvious how to proceed, and the diagnosis is borderline. On the whole, it is best to explain this to the patient and, if it is decided to proceed, change the method where one does not prove successful. Be honest with the patient; not all cases will respond and there is no reward for anyone in unsuccessful treatment.

PREVENTION

It is important to discover amblyopia or the factors which may cause it, at as early an age as possible. A great deal can be done in the prevention of amblyopia if it is discovered by regular eye examination in early childhood. This is particularly true of those types of amblyopia in which refractive error plays a large part in the cause: in accommodative squint, in anisometropic and astigmatic amblyopia. The children who are at greatest risk are those whose parents or brothers and sisters have amblyopia and/or squints. It should be explained to any young adult with these conditions that their children could have similar problems, and that early eye examination is strongly advised and should be repeated at regular intervals to prevent any loss of vision developing. Similarly, the parents of children with amblyopia or squint should be routinely advised to have the patient's brothers or sisters checked.

SPECTACLE CORRECTION

A clear retinal image is required for the normal development of acuity. Where the patient is under the age of 10 years and the acuity of the amblyopic eye is 6/24 or better, improvement is likely with the spectacle correction alone in those cases where the refractive error is a factor in the cause of the amblyopia. Glasses should be worn for 6–8 weeks, to allow the maximum improvement to occur before any other types of treatment are undertaken.

In other cases, glasses are indicated where they improve the clarity of the retinal images, balance the accommodative effort between the two eyes, or where they reduce the angle of a squint.

The prescribing of glasses for squint is described in Chapter 15.

OCCLUSION

In the general treatment of amblyopia, occlusion of the non-amblyopic eye, 'direct occlusion', is a long established method and has proved to produce good results in many cases (Pickwell, 1977). The usual method is total occlusion, which tries to ensure that no light enters the eye and the amblyopic eye is brought into use. The most effective device is an adhesive patch which covers the eye and extends a little over the orbit margins. A smaller piece of gauze or lint in the centre prevents adhesion to the lids. Plastic, rubber or felt cup devices are also made to fit between the eye and the spectacles. These do not provide such total occlusion and a young child can soon learn to peep over them. The occlusion is usually full time; that is worn all day, only coming off when the patient is in bed.

When occlusion is thought to be the best procedure, it is maintained for 2 or 3 months in order to get the maximum response. Weekly checks of the acuity of both eyes are carried out during this time. Usually no marked improvement is found for the first several weeks, and if there is no response after 5 weeks, it is unlikely that an improvement will occur. If the patient is over 3 years of age, any loss of acuity in the occluded eye will return when the occlusion treatment ceases. Under 3 years, the occluder, or patch, should be worn over the non-amblyopic eye for 3 days and then changed to the amblyopic eye for 1 day to allow the development of the non-amblyopic eye. As a means of therapy, occlusion of the amblyopic eye, 'inverse occlusion', does not seem to be effective (von Noorden, 1965). Even where there is eccentric fixation, direct occlusion is recommended.

During a period of occlusion, the treatment can be made more effective by asking the patient to undertake a definitive visual task for several 10-minute periods each day, to interest the patient and stimulate vision in the amblyopic eye. These should be presented to younger children as games or competitions. For example, children can be asked to write as many words as possible on a square the size of a postage stamp, or see how small they can write in copying out a poem. Other exercises can easily be devised (see *Figure 11.3*). A patient can be asked to read through a passage of news print and neatly cross out every letter e. Video games have been devised for use as an exercise for amblyopia. In carrying out such exercises, care must be taken to ensure that the patient is working at the limit of acuity by maintaining a proper working distance and not allowing the eyes to move very close to the page. The distance should also be monitored when the patient is watching television or playing television games.

When the acuity ceases to improve, the occluder may be removed in the case of the refractive amblyopes. Where there is a squint, the next step in the total treatment needs to be considered. If the occluder is removed and the patient left with a squint, it is likely that the amblyopia will return or that the patient will experience diplopia. If single binocular vision cannot be restored at once, it will be necessary to replace the total occlusion with some form of partial occlusion of the non-amblyopic eye. This is done by sticking on the back of the spectacle lens a patch of Sellotape, Scotch tape or other semi-transparent material, which reduces the acuity of the non-amblyopic eye to a little below that of the squinting eye. This will ensure that the acuity does not deteriorate while other treatment is proceeding, and is said to help in overcoming any abnormal retinal correspondence.

In refractive amblyopia, the improvement may not be maintained in patients under 10 years of age, and occlusion may have to be resumed. Sometimes simultaneous vision exercises such as those described in Chapter 8 for the treatment

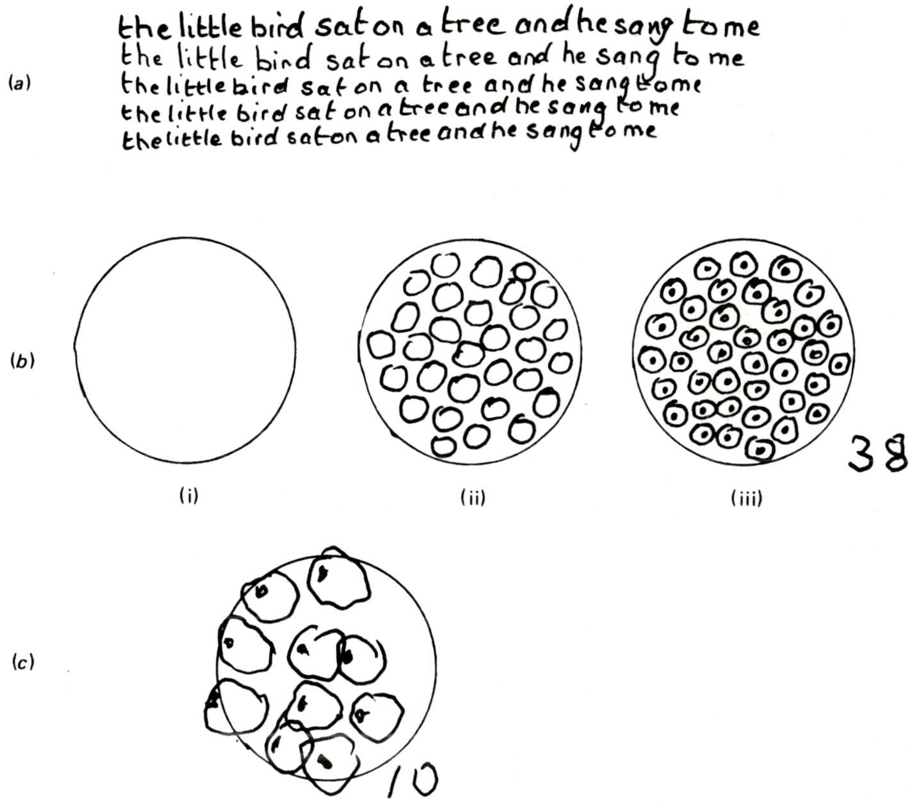

Figure 11.3. Examples of fine detail exercises for amblyopia when the non-amblyopic eye is occluded. (a) Small writing; note that there are no lines, and the patient is asked to write as close to the preceding line as possible without overlap. (b) 'Frog spawn': (i) stage 1, a circle produced by drawing round a coin; (ii) stage 2, the patient has filled the circle with small rings; (iii) stage 3, the patient has added a dot in the middle of each ring and counted the number, (38). (c) An example from a patient with poor acuity and eccentric localization. Note that there is a tendency to localize too far to the left–shown at both stages 2 and 3

of central suppression will help to maintain good acuity without resuming occlusion. Sellotape, to reduce the acuity of the better eye, may also help in these cases.

In those patients where difficulty is likely to be experienced in persuading them to wear the occluder, a trial period of partial occlusion or inverse occlusion may help. Full total occlusion may then be more acceptable to the patient.

Part-time occlusion can be considered where full-time occlusion is inappropriate due to the very reduced acuity, or where it would be dangerous to occlude full time.

SUPPRESSION TREATMENT

Suppression treatment as a means of improving the acuity in anisometropic amblyopia can be very successful as an alternative to occlusion. Although occlusion is sometimes necessary, it is not always the preferred method: if good binocular vision is the ultimate aim, perhaps covering one eye is not always the best way to start! In cases where there is no squint, and the effect of the spectacle correction has been tried for 6–8 weeks, further improvement in acuity can sometimes be produced by exercises which ensure that the amblyopic eye is used with its fellow. It is useful to investigate the depth and extent of the suppression, and where it appears appropriate to give treatment for any suppression found. Exercises described in Chapter 12 may be required, but often the simpler treatment outlined for suppression in heterophoria in Chapter 8 will help considerably. Most teenage patients would prefer this approach to having to wear an occluder (Pickwell and Jenkins, 1983).

PHYSIOLOGICAL DIPLOPIA

In some cases, physiological diplopia methods can be used as an alternative to occlusion in convergent squint. The method is simple to understand, but in practice it may require a lot of patient supervision. A near-vision fixation distance is found where the visual axes cross in convergent squint, and an appreciation of physiological diplopia is used to encourage the use of binocular vision. This brings the amblyopic eye into use with the other eye at one fixation distance, and results in an improvement in acuity over several weeks.

The difficulty in applying this method is usually in the early stages. In theory, it is not difficult to see that there is a point in front of the eyes of a patient with convergent squint where the visual axes cross and that an object placed there ought to have a foveal image in both eyes; the object is being fixed binocularly. In practice, this can be found by using the cover test and moving the object closer or further away until no squint movement is seen. Where the patient increases the angle of deviation as the object is moved towards the eyes (the convergence excess element), this can sometimes be inhibited by explaining to the patient that the eye is turning inwards too much and encouraging less convergence. This may take time.

With some patients, convergence needs to be inhibited by positive spherical additions. When binocular fixation of the object has been achieved, the patient is encouraged to see a second object in physiological diplopia. This should be introduced at a greater distance than the fixation. Its image will then fall on the nasal retina in the area where there are likely to be binocular sensory adaptations which developed in the squint (see *Figure 10.1*). With further encouragement, appreciation of physiological diplopia of the second object can be seen, while fixation of the first is maintained. A week of home exercise supervised by a parent should consolidate this. The parent may be taught how to apply the cover test to check that fixation has been maintained. The patient then progresses to wire reading, which is described in Chapter 8. It should be checked that the reading material is in a print size that is within the limits of the patient's acuity for near vision.

This method is appropriate only to angles of squint less than 12^{Δ} or in which it can be reduced to this by the spectacle correction. It requires a high degree of interest and co-operation. The starting acuity should be 6/24 or better, and in some cases can go on improving for several months if the method is successful in establishing binocular vision for close work. The method is further described in Chapter 12 in relation to its use in the treatment of binocular sensory adaptations.

RED FILTER OCCLUSION

This method is said to be useful in the treatment of eccentric fixation for younger children, but it has also been used in other amblyopia cases. It consists of inverse occlusion (of the amblyopic eye) for most of the day, but for a short period of 10 minutes, increasing to half a day, the occluder is changed to the other eye and a dark red filter (Wratten filter No. 92) is placed before the amblyopic eye. With this filter and the occluder in place before the other eye, the patient is encouraged to use the amblyopic eye as much as possible. The evidence of clinical evaluations of this method is very conflicting, and the underlying theory behind it is doubtful (Pickwell, 1977). Some practitioners have reported good results, and in some cases using much lighter filters which are very much less monochromatic than the Wratten No. 92.

AFTER-IMAGE TRANSFER METHOD

A central after-image is created in the dominant eye, and transferred to the amblyopic eye as described later in the chapter. The patient is then asked to try to locate the after-image at the point of fixation, and to see smaller fixation letters. The procedure is repeated when the after-image fades, and the acuity is measured after several repeats (Caloroso, 1972; Mallett, 1975).

Although originally advocated for eccentric fixation, the method can produce improvement in other amblyopia cases. It appears that the best results are obtained when the starting acuity is 6/24 or better, and in those cases when the binocular vision and acuity had deteriorated following previous improvement achieved by other orthoptic procedures (Jenkins, Pickwell and Sheridan, 1979).

PENALIZATION

The method consists of maintaining cycloplegia of both eyes by a weekly application of 1% atropine ointment, and providing the non-amblyopic eye with a reading addition: +3 D sphere. This allows the use of the amblyopic eye for distance vision, and the other for near work. It is claimed that the co-operation of the patient is assured, as there is no occluder to peep round, no exercises to be skipped and the glasses must be worn if the patient wishes to see clearly. However, it will be appreciated that where the acuity in the amblyopic eye is worse than 6/36, the patient may have better acuity with the other eye by looking over the glasses or by taking them off. This will depend on the refractive error (Gregorson, Pontoppidas and Rindziunki, 1974). An alternative method is to have the reading addition in the amblyopic eye and a normal correction in the other (Dale, 1982).

FOGGING METHOD

In this approach, the non-amblyopic eye is fogged for distance vision by an extra positive sphere, +2 D or +3 D, which serves as a reading addition for near. This is a less dramatic way of producing a similar situation to drug penalization – clear distance vision in the amblyopic eye and near vision with the other. These glasses may be worn all the time, or as a second pair which is worn in the evenings each day while watching television. In a partially accommodative squint, this method assists in further reducing the angle.

EUTHYSCOPE

A special ophthalmoscope is used to centre a wide ring after-image on the fovea of the amblyopic eye. The fovea itself is spared the after-image, while the surrounding retina, including the eccentrically fixing area, is 'desensitized' by the after-image. The patient is then asked to look at individual letters in decreasing sizes with true foveal fixation. To the patient, the appearance of the after-image is that of a ring, in the centre of the field, and with a hole in the middle in which the letter can be seen. The after-image includes the eccentric area otherwise used for fixation, so that it cannot be used during this method of treatment. The method requires the use of a mydriatic for most patients, and daily treatment is recommended. While the ophthalmoscope is being correctly centred by the practitioner to ensure an exact central after-image, the patient steadies both eyes by fixing a light spot across the room with the other eye. This is seen in a small mirror, supported on a headband if necessary to ensure that the practitioner's head does not get in the way. A number of instruments have been designed for this method. They include the euthyscope, and the Keeler Projectoscope.

This method requires a lot of practitioner time, and is very tiring for the patient. To be effective, it needs to be rigorously applied. It has never proved very easy or popular. There is no clear evidence of the success of this method.

HAIDINGER'S BRUSHES

Central fixation may be encouraged by asking the patient to see Haidinger's brushes by the methods described later in the chapter. In the first place, an empty bright blue field of rotating polarized light is used, and then a fixation letter or other target is introduced.

ROTATING GRATING

In recent years, a method has been suggested in which the patient is required to look at a rotating grating of black and white lines for a few minutes, and to maintain clear vision of the lines – the CAM disc method (Banks *et al.*, 1978). This method has not been shown to produce good results (Douthwaite *et al.*, 1981). Several recent studies indicate that it produces the same results as occlusion, which may also be required. It is a little more effective in anisometropic amblyopia than in strabismic (Gunnar and Samuelson, 1983; Nyman *et al.*, 1983).

References

BANKS, R. V., CAMPBELL, F. W., HESS, R. and WATSON, P. G. (1978). A new treatment for amblyopia. *British Orthoptic Journal*, **35,** 1–12

BROCKBANK, G. and DOWNEY, R. (1959). Measurement of eccentric fixation by the Bjerrum screen. *British Journal of Ophthalmology*, **45,** 461–465

CALOROSO, E. (1972). After-image transfer: a therapeutic procedure for amblyopia. *American Journal of Optometry*, **49,** 65–69

CHAVASSE, F. B. (1939). *Worth's Squint*, 7th edn. Baillière Tindall, London

DALE, R. T. (1982). *Fundamentals of Ocular Motility and Strabismus*. Grune & Stratton, New York, p. 156

DOUTHWAITE, W. A., JENKINS, T. C. A., PICKWELL, L. D. and SHERIDAN, M. (1981). The treatment of amblyopia by the rotating grating method. *Ophthalmic and Physiological Optics*, **1,** 97–106

FLOM, M. C. and WEYMOUTH, F. W. (1961). Centricity of Maxwell's spot in strabismus and amblyopia. *Archives of Ophthalmology*, **66,** 260

GREGORSON, E., PONTOPPIDAS, M. and RINDZIUNKI, E. (1974). Drug penalisation treatment of amblyopia. *Acta Ophthalmologica*, **52,** 60–66

GUNNAR, L. and SAMUELSON, B. (1983). Amblyopia in 4 year old children treated with grating stimulation and full-time occlusion; a comparative study. *British Journal of Ophthalmology*, **67,** 181–190

JENKINS, T. C. A., PICKWELL, L. D. and SHERIDAN, M. (1979). After-image transfer – evaluation of short-term treatment. *British Journal of Physiological Optics*, **33**(3), 33–37

LINKSZ, A. (1952). *Physiology of the Eye*, vol. 2, *Vision*. Grune & Stratton, New York, pp.534–541

LYLE, K. T. and WYBAR, K. C. (1967). *Practical Orthoptics in the Treatment of Squint*. Lewis, London, pp. 82–83

MALLETT, R. J. F. (1975). Using after-images in the investigation and treatment of strabismus. *The Ophthalmic Optician*, **15,** 727–729

NOORDEN, G. K., VON (1965). Occlusion therapy in amblyopia with eccentric fixation. *Archives of Ophthalmology*, **73,** 776

NOORDEN, G. K., VON (1974). Factors involved in the production of amblyopia. *British Journal of Ophthalmology*, **38,** 158–164

NYMAN, K. G., SINGH, G., RYDBERG, A. and FORDANDER, M. (1983). Controlled study comparing CAM treatment with occlusion therapy. *British Journal of Ophthalmology*, **67,** 178–180

PICKWELL, L. D. (1977). The management of amblyopia: a review. *The Ophthalmic Optician*, **17,** 743–745

PICKWELL, L. D. and JENKINS, T. C. A. (1982). Orthoptic treatment in teenage patients. *Ophthalmic and Physiological Optics*, **2**(3), 221–225

PICKWELL, L. D. and JENKINS, T. C. A. (1983). Response to amblyopia treatment. *Australian Journal of Optometry*, **66**(1), 29–33

12

Suppression and abnormal retinal correspondence

Suppression and abnormal retinal correspondence are adaptations in the visual sensory mechanisms which occur in squint. They develop usually before the visual system has become firmly established; that is, before the age of about 6 years. These adaptations have been reviewed in general outline in Chapter 10, and are further described in this chapter with particular reference to the clinical investigation and treatment. As explained in Chapter 10, the two binocular adaptations are interrelated and usually both occur in small angle squints. In squints over 25^{Δ}, suppression seems to dominate.

Suppression

If the corresponding retinal points in the two eyes are presented with differing stimuli, the neural signal from one of the retinal elements is suppressed. This can be demonstrated in normal subjects by the phenomenon called 'retinal rivalry'. This is seen when two different images are presented to the eyes in a stereoscope. A changing pattern of intermittent suppression of retinal areas occurs as one or other of each pair of retinal elements is suppressed. Which one of these corresponding retinal elements is suppressed will depend on the relative strength or degree of interest of the two stimuli. When they are equal, the ocular dominance may be a factor, but in normal subjects there is a rhythm of change in the mosaic of alternating areas between the two eyes.

In squint, the deviation will mean that corresponding points will not receive the same image, and this will be a constant factor. The result is a loss of the rhythm of retinal rivalry over an area of the retina extending from the centre nasally in convergent squint (see *Figure 10.1*). As indicated in Chapter 10, suppression seems to be concerned with the perception of form, and is an inhibition of the '*x*-cell' system. Abnormal retinal correspondence is concerned with visual direction of images, and is a loss of resolution in the '*y*-cell' system due to an abnormal increase in the convergence of nerve paths caused by the neural elements being connected with each other at some level. Abnormal retinal correspondence is discussed further later in this chapter.

In a unilateral squint, the suppression will always be in the same eye; the squinting eye. In an alternating squint, the eye which happens to be deviated at the

Smc

time will be suppressed. It must be emphasized that suppression is an anomaly of binocular vision. In monocular vision, there will be no inhibition of vision of this kind, whichever eye is unoccluded. Indeed, alternating squints can have full acuity in both eyes when they are examined monocularly. In unilateral squints, suppression is usually accompanied by amblyopia in the squinting eye.

Where the squint has been present from an early age, before 3 years, the cortical cells receiving images from both eyes, the 'binocularly driven' cells, do not seem to develop. The earlier the onset of the squint, the fewer binocularly driven cells there seem to be. If a squint with early onset is left untreated until after the age of 5 or 6 years, integration of the images from the two eyes (fusion) may never be possible. The lack of the fusion ability means that the motor deviation will always be present, as there can be no binocular lock to maintain straightness of the eyes, and the patient will have suppression. If this should be treated, diplopia is most likely to result.

Investigation

The investigation of suppression consists largely of determining its depth and the extent of the retinal area concerned. Both factors may be affected by the spectacle correction: a clear retinal image may help to overcome suppression. If the glasses reduce the angle of the squint, the depth and extent of the suppression may also be reduced.

DEPTH OF SUPPRESSION

There are a number of clinical methods which will help in the investigation of the depth of the suppression. In those cases where the suppression can easily be overcome, shallow suppression, it is more likely that treatment will be successful. However, it should also be remembered that, in shallow suppression, prescribing glasses is more likely to cause diplopia. This is desirable if the angle of the deviation can then be treated, but care needs to be taken in other cases – see also the later section on management.

Infinity balance or septum test

The details of this test are described in Chapter 3 (see *Figure 3.1*). It can be useful in the investigation of suppression in anisometropia or in some small angle squints, as well as in suppression accompanying heterophoria. Suppression may be overcome on the septum test either spontaneously or with the encouragement of momentary occlusion of the non-suppressing eye. Where this occurs, shallow suppression is indicated. Where the acuity of the amblyopic eye is less than 6/12, larger letters than the standard LF must be used.

Filter bar method

This consists of finding the depth of filter held before the non-suppressing eye which will overcome the suppression. The filters are used in the form of a filter bar or ladder: this is a series of filters of increasing absorption mounted in a continuous strip so that they can be introduced before the eye one after the other (see *Figure 12.1*). Two types of filter bar are available. One has neutral density filters, and the other red filters of increasing depth.

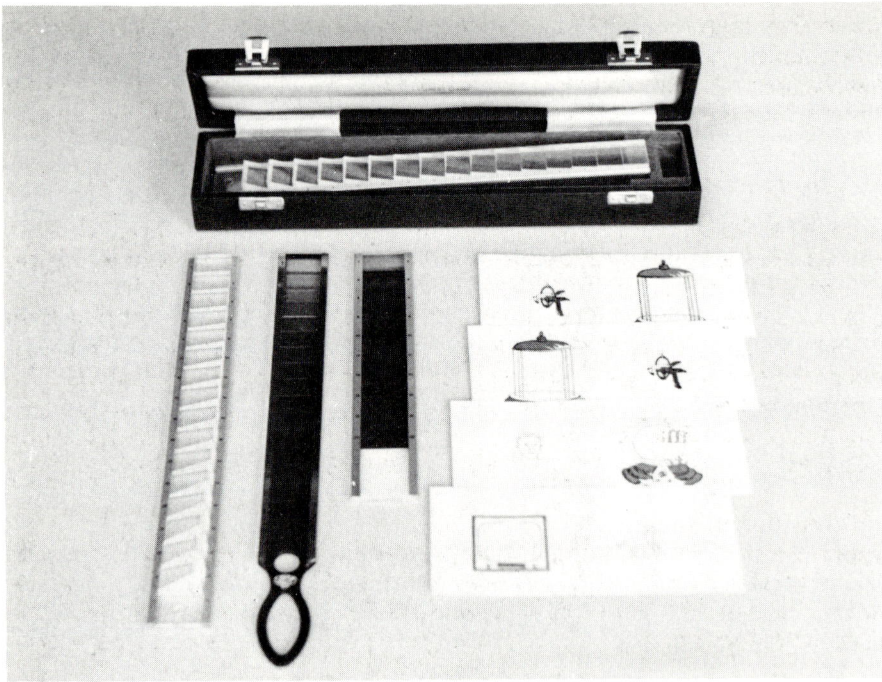

Figure 12.1. Vertical prism bar (top); horizontal prism bar (left); Bagolini red filter bar and a Mallett neutral density filter bar (centre); Bradford stereoscope cards, A series, for simultaneous vision (right)

The method is to ask the patient to look at a small spot of light and to introduce the filter bar before the non-suppressing eye, beginning with the lightest filter. As the darker filters are moved before the eye, the retinal illuminance will be decreased until the patient sees two lights. The depth of filter used will be a measure of the suppression.

Synoptophore

The depth of suppression can also be estimated by the size and brightness of pictures of the synoptophore slides. Large brightly coloured pictures before the squinting eye overcome suppression more readily, so that a hierarchy of slides can be established, and patients can be classified as having suppression with one slide and not with another. 'Fusion' slides with most of the picture common to both eyes are more likely to be suppressed than 'simultaneous vision' slides which have a quite different picture for each eye.

Stereoscope method

Stereoscope cards can be graded in the same way as synoptophore slides described above. Examples of these are shown in *Figure 12.1*. The cards are printed with the larger picture before the right eye, and another card with it before the left. The larger picture is first presented to the suppressing eye, and if both pictures can be seen, the smaller picture is then given to the suppressing eye to see if this is seen or suppressed.

More shallow suppression can also be judged by the size of type suppressed when using the 'interrupted passages' cards shown in *Figure 8.1*.

In squint cases, the variable prism stereoscope is usually employed for this type of investigation, as the prisms allow adjustment to the angle of squint.

EXTENT OF SUPPRESSION SCOTOMA

Sensory changes in two retinal areas are required to avoid confusion and diplopia – in the foveal area and in the peripheral area which receives the image of the object of the patient's attention. The usual description, therefore, is that of two suppression scotomas requiring some form of binocular scotometry to demonstrate them. They are not monocular field losses, but require some form of binocular haploscopic device which will allow fixation with one eye while the visibility of a target moved in the field of the other eye is plotted. In long-standing squint, the two suppression scotomas may be so large that they join each other and produce one large elliptical scotoma. They are also more extensive in large angle squints.

Suppression scotometry

The patient is seated in the normal position in front of a Bjerrum screen. A small mirror is mounted at an angle of about 45° before the fixing eye, so that the screen is occluded from this eye but it can fix a small marker at the side of the patient and at the same distance as the screen (see *Figure 12.2*). Both eyes are kept open

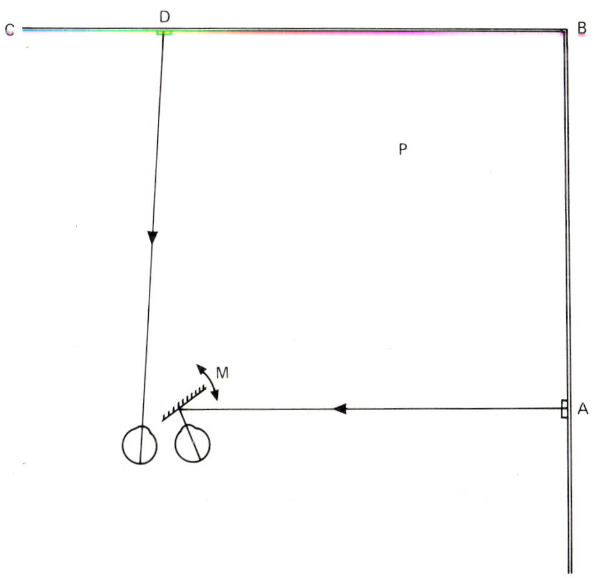

Figure 12.2. Suppression scotometry with the single mirror haploscope. The patient is seated in the corner of a room at equal distance from both the walls, AB and BC. A fixation object, A, is seen on wall AB in a mirror which can be rotated about a vertical axis, but makes an angle of about 45° to the patient's line of sight. Targets can be moved on the wall, BC, in the field of the other eye, and the patient is asked to report when one or the other of the targets is suppressed, so that the suppression area can be plotted. The single mirror haploscope can also be used for the treatment of abnormal retinal correspondence, and it has been used with fusion targets on the walls for vergence exercises by rotating the mirror. The practitioner sitting at P can observe the patient's eyes without obscuring the targets

throughout the test. Bjerrum screen targets are moved from the centre of the screen until they are reported as being seen by the patient; that is, until they are outside the suppression area. This is repeated for all directions until the full size and shape of the scotoma has been plotted. The size of the scotoma will vary with the size of target used. A large target is likely to reveal a small central scotoma, but a smaller target, 2 mm, will extend into the area of abnormal correspondence and will not be distinguished by the patient as separate from the fixation spot.

Prism bar method

The patient fixes a spotlight with the dominant eye, while the prism bar is moved before the suppressing eye. When the image of the spot has moved off the suppression scotoma, the patient will report double vision. If the starting point is taken as the prism power which relieves the angle of the squint shown by the cover test, the angular extent of the suppression scotoma from the fovea can be determined. The vertical prism bar will give the vertical extent. A red filter may be used before one eye, but this will decrease the size of the scotoma.

Synoptophore method

The horizontal size of the suppression scotoma can be measured for a particular pair of synoptophore slides by moving the tube before the suppressing eye across the field and noting where the image disappears and reappears. The patient maintains central fixation with the other eye throughout. The size of the scotoma will depend on the particular slides used, so that this needs to be standardized by using the same pair for all patients. Usually, slides specially designed for diagnosis are used. These may consist of a small fixation object for one eye and a circle or square of about 10° angular size for the deviating eye.

Evaluation

The evaluation of the investigation of suppression in squint has to be considered together with the assessment of all the other factors present in any particular case. It will be appreciated that if factors such as the patient's age, duration for which the squint has been present, degree of co-operation likely and the other factors are favourable, the treatment of the suppression will be more likely to be successful. Considering the suppression alone, the deeper the suppression and the greater the extent across the retina, the more difficult it will be to treat.

It must also be remembered that suppression is an adaptation to the squint. It is therefore not desirable to treat it, unless there is a very good chance that the deviation can also be eliminated. If the sensory adaptations to the squint are treated but the squint remains, the patient will be troubled by confusion and diplopia.

Where suppression accompanies anisometropia, there is less danger of producing troublesome diplopia. In such cases, the treatment of suppression can take place at the same time as treatment of any amblyopia. This treatment will be preceded by prescribing a suitable spectacle correction.

Management

The general aim of treatment of suppression is to encourage the patient to become aware of the suppressed image, and then to integrate it correctly with the image from the other eye. Both aspects of this are essential for normal binocular vision. In order to avoid strengthening abnormal retinal correspondence, it is important that method of treatment ensures simultaneous stimulation of the foveal areas of both eyes, or of other pairs of normally corresponding points. Simultaneous stimulation of normally corresponding points requires that the angle of the squint must be relieved during treatment. This can be done by the glasses in fully accommodative squint, and in other squints by prisms, or the use of a stereoscope or synoptophore set at the angle of the squint. In some convergent squint, a position in front of the eyes where the visual axes interesect may be found: bifoveal images of an object placed at this position can be a good starting point.

It is important to take precautions against making the abnormal correspondence more deeply ingrained. The best precaution is to consider the treatment of the suppression and the abnormal correspondence together. It must be emphasized that it is not sufficient to obtain simultaneous vision of any kind, but the aim is simultaneous vision of normally corresponding areas.

One or more of the following methods may be useful in the management of suppression in squinting patients or in anisometropia.

SYNOPTOPHORE

At one time this was the principal instrument used in the treatment of squint, and is still used in some clinics. A brighter, more highly coloured slide before the suppressing eye is used to encourage simultaneous vision. The slide before the suppressing eye is changed for one with less colour or smaller picture size until suppression occurs. The patient is then asked to try to overcome the suppression by seeing the picture for both eyes at the same time, for example, the soldier seen by one eye inside the sentry-box seen with the other eye. When the suppression intervenes, the picture can be moved slightly by shaking the tube back and forward a few degrees, or by tapping the slide extraction lever to make the slide jump up and down.

A 'chasing' exercise can also be used: the practitioner moves one tube about 10° and the patient is asked to move the other to regain superimposition of the pictures; the sentry in the box. When this has been done, the first tube is moved again, and so on. The tube before the suppressing eye can be flashed on and off to attract the attention of the suppressing eye. It must be emphasized, however, that each time the patient reports that both pictures can be seen, a check must be made to ensure that this is at the correct angle of squint; that there is really bifoveal vision. This check can be made by switching off the tube before the dominant eye, while watching that there is no movement of the other eye. This is the equivalent of performing the cover test to check for the presence of a squint.

RED FILTER METHOD

The patient has a red filter before the dominant eye, and is asked to trace a picture on tracing paper using a red pencil or ball-point pen. Through the red filter, the page will appear to be red, so that the patient's own drawing in red cannot be seen against it with the dominant eye and the suppressing eye has to be used. Younger patients can be encouraged to sort coloured beads, and in order to do this the suppressing eye must be used, as the true colours cannot be seen through the red filter. Before using this method it is necessary to ensure that there is good monocular acuity, and that in squint the possibility of abnormal correspondence has been eliminated.

STEREOSCOPES

In large angle squints, over 10^{Δ}, a variable prism stereoscope is used and the prism power adjusted to compensate for the angle of the squint. For smaller angle squints, it may be possible to get superimposition of the pictures with a Holmes stereoscope by adjusting the card distance. The difficulty with either type of stereoscope is being sure that bifoveal vision is being stimulated. Some instruments are designed so that the cover test can be performed while the patient looks through the lenses. With some patients, the possibility of abnormal retinal correspondence can be eliminated, but with many others the danger that there may be stimulation of non-corresponding points is present, and this method is not appropriate. It is better not to do the exercise than to deepen the abnormal correspondence.

Where this method is appropriate, cards should be used that require the patient to see at the limit of the acuity of the amblyopic eye. The smaller the detail seen, the less is the chance of abnormal correspondence. The Bradford stereoscope cards, F series (see *Figure 8.1*), are suitable, and the card is found with a type size which can just be read by the amblyopic eye. The method is described in Chapter 8.

PHYSIOLOGICAL DIPLOPIA

This method is appropriate in those cases when a point can be found where the visual axes cross in front of the eyes in convergent squint. The details of the method are described in Chapter 11, and are further developed in a later section of this chapter on the management of abnormal retinal correspondence. The advantage of the method, when it is possible, is that the cover test can be undertaken at any time to ensure bifoveal fixation.

It will be apparent that in all squint the possibility of stimulating non-corresponding points is present with all of these methods, and very great care has to be exercised to ensure that this does not happen. It means very careful supervision. To begin with, most of the binocular treatment should be given in the consulting room where it can be overseen by the practitioner. Home treatment in the early stages should be confined to the monocular types of treatment for amblyopia. As the case progresses, some home treatment can be given by carefully instructing the parent on how to check for simultaneous macular vision; a simple explanation of the cover test check may suffice. Patients should, however, be seen at very frequent intervals – every few days – at this stage.

The methods described above, however, are certainly appropriate to suppression which may accompany anisometropia with no squint, as it is unlikely that there will be abnormal retinal correspondence in these cases.

Abnormal retinal correspondence

As previously explained, abnormal retinal correspondence is an adaptation in the sensory visual system which occurs in the interest of avoiding diplopia in a squinting patient. It is present during the patient's everyday vision, but normal correspondence may return in some of the special conditions of investigative tests. The likelihood of normal correspondence being temporarily re-established during investigation will depend on the conditions under which the test is performed.

Some conditions favour normal correspondence and some abnormal. If the conditions favour normal correspondence, but the result of the test shows it to be abnormal, it is likely that this abnormality is firmly established and is less likely to respond to treatment. It is therefore important to understand the factors that favour normal correspondence. Before discussing the factors, a description of the tests used in the investigation of retinal correspondence will be given.

Investigation of retinal correspondence

There are several methods currently used for the investigation of retinal correspondence. Because the correspondence may be normal with some methods and abnormal using others, due to the change in the conditions of the test, it is necessary to have more than one method available. This allows a better assessment of the correspondence to be made, and will help in determining the prognosis. One method is not necessarily more reliable than others, but when several methods are used which have different conditions, a better picture of the intensity to which the abnormality has developed is obtained. Some of the following methods can be recommended.

STRIATE LENS METHOD

The striate lens is a plano trial-case lens which has a fine grating of lines ruled on it (Bagolini, 1971). This allows the patient to see through the lens with very little disturbance of normal vision, but when looking at a spot of light, the lens produces a faint streak crossing the light. In unilateral squint, one lens can be used before the deviated eye to produce a vertical streak rather like a 'see-through' Maddox rod, while the patient looks at a spot of light with both eyes open. If the streak appears to pass through the spot of light, harmonious abnormal correspondence is demonstrated. A suppression area may result in a gap in the central part of the streak, but the patient may be able to report that the ends of it can be seen in line with the spot.

In alternating deviations, it is usually necessary to use a striate lens before both eyes, so that they produce streaks at 45° in one eye and 135° in the other. When the two streaks appear to pass through the light spot, harmonious abnormal correspondence is demonstrated.

If the streak does not pass through the spot, either normal correspondence or inharmonious abnormal correspondence is shown, depending on whether the angular separation of the spot and the streak is the same as the angle of the deviation. With inharmonious abnormal retinal correspondence, the angle of the separation between the spot and the streak, the angle of diplopia, is less than the angle of the squint.

A filter bar can be used before the squinting eye to help in the assessment of any abnormal correspondence. If the patient has predominantly normal correspondence, but will revert to abnormal during the everyday circumstances when the adaptation is needed to alleviate diplopia, a pale filter will cause diplopia or suppression. In cases of more firmly established abnormal correspondence, a more dense filter will be required before suppression or normal correspondence intervenes.

Several kinds of Bagolini striate lenses can be obtained, some giving more obvious streaks than others. The more faint the streak produced, the more likely it is that abnormal correspondence and suppression will occur, as there is very little disturbance of the patient's habitual vision.

SYNOPTOPHORE METHOD

This instrument is still used for the measurement of angles of squint and the investigation of correspondence. Again, the results can be very confusing unless great care is taken over the method and the routine employed. It is important to distinguish between the habitual angle and the total angle of the squint, otherwise the total angle may be measured, and when the subjective angle is compared the eyes will have returned to their habitual position and inharmonious abnormal correspondence is incorrectly diagnosed. The eyes must be kept under observation all the time, so that their position can be checked objectively by reference to the corneal reflections of the light from the synoptophore tubes.

Use simultaneous vision slides; for example, a circle before one eye and a square for the other. A central fixation mark on each slide should allow as precise fixation as the acuity will permit. The patient is asked to fix with the dominant eye. Then the tube before this eye is momentarily switched off, while the practitioner watches the movement of the other eye in taking up fixation. The tube before the deviated eye is then moved so as to make this movement unnecessary. This is repeated until no movement occurs. The angle of the tubes then shows the habitual angle of the squint. If the patient now sees the two fixation objects in the same position, normal correspondence is demonstrated by this method.

The illumination of the two tubes is then alternated, and the patient asked to look from the square to the circle and back as each is illuminated. Any further deviation which occurs is neutralized by moving the tubes. This will give the total, or objective, angle of the squint. Continue to alternate the illumination and ask the patient if the square and circle appear in the same place, or if there is any apparent jump – phi movement.

The angles measured by this method may be more convergent than those found with other methods, due to proximal convergence. The Stanworth modification to the synoptophore relieves this proximal convergence (Stanworth, 1958). The mirrors of a standard instrument are replaced in this model by semi-silvered mirrors, so that when the illumination of a tube is reduced the patient can see through the mirror and fix an object across the room. This also removes some of the artificiality of the instrument, as the patient is fixing a real object rather than an image. The combination of these factors has given results which show that most patients have harmonious rather than inharmonious abnormal retinal correspondence, which is also the case with the striate lens method.

RED FILTER DIPLOPIA METHOD

In this method, the patient is asked to look at a spot of light with both eyes, while a red filter is held before the squinting eye. This filter helps to overcome the suppression and allows the patient to see two lights – a red and a white one. If the spot is still suppressed, a vertical prism is introduced before one eye to move the image above or below the suppression scotoma. The power of the prism, 6^Δ–15^Δ, will depend on the size of the scotoma. When both the red and white images of the spot are seen, the patient is asked to report if they are in vertical alignment or if one is further to the right or left of the other. If they are aligned one immediately above the other, abnormal correspondence is indicated. Otherwise, there is either normal correspondence or inharmonious abnormal correspondence, depending on the degree of horizontal separation compared to the angle of the squint.

A relieving prism can be held before the eye so that there is a central image in both eyes. In normal correspondence, the patient should then report vertical alignment.

AFTER-IMAGE METHOD

In this method, each eye in turn takes up fixation of a bright light, while the other eye is occluded. This produces a central foveal after-image. If there is normal correspondence, the two after-images will be seen in the same direction, but if the foveal areas no longer correspond, the after-images will appear separated. It will be noted that once the after-images are created, the visual direction in which they are seen relative to each other will not be affected by the position of the eyes or the angle of the squint, but only by the retinal correspondence. Very occasionally, a convergent squint may have abnormal correspondence for distance, but not at near vision, and sometimes in intermittent divergent squint the abnormal correspondence is present when the eye is deviated, but not when both are straight. Otherwise, the correspondence is not changed by the movements of the eyes.

If the sensory adaptations to the squint are very marked and long standing, there may be some difficulty in the patient seeing the after-image. The following routine is suggested. Use a photographic flashgun with the front masked so that it produces a line flash with a short bar across the centre to act as a fixation point and to mark the fovea on the after-image. The patient fixes first with the dominant eye, the flashgun being held horizontally, and the gun is fired. Then the patient fixes the centre mark with the usually squinting eye, while the flashgun is held upright to produce a vertical line after-image. The patient then closes both eyes until both after-images can be seen. If the foveal centres of these images coincide so as to form a cross, normal correspondence is present under these conditions. If the vertical after-image cuts the horizontal one to one side of the centre or is separated horizontally from the horizontal line, abnormal correspondence is indicated. At this stage, the patient is asked to open the eyes and look at a plain surface. Negative after-images are then produced, and their relative positions can be judged under these slightly different conditions. A fixation point can then be provided for the dominant eye, and a third assessment of their relative positions made. With the eyes closed, the dissociation between the eyes is almost complete. When a fixation point is provided, the dissociation is less and the conditions are a little closer to the patient's habitual vision.

If a flashgun is not available, the patient can be asked to look at a suitable light bulb, fixing the top for 7 seconds with the dominant eye first, and then the bottom for 10 seconds with the other eye. It is important that a check is made to ensure that the eye maintains steady fixation. The after-images will consist of two bulb shapes, one higher that the other, and their relative positions can be judged to assess the correspondence.

It will be clear that, in patients with eccentric fixation, the after-image will be created at the eccentrically fixing area and not at the fovea. Abnormal correspondence is an anomaly of squint and most squinting eyes have eccentric fixation. This will mean that the angle of eccentric fixation needs to be determined before proceeding to the after-image test. If this angle is the same, or nearly the same, as the angle of the squint, the separation of the after-images will not be found when there is abnormal correspondence. This is true of microsquint (see Chapter 13).

VISUAL CONDITIONS AFFECTING RETINAL CORRESPONDENCE

The foregoing description of methods of investigating retinal correspondence shows that the visual conditions of the various tests differ, and as a result some tests will show normal correspondence and others abnormal. There are five interrelated factors which determine the visual conditions, and these are considered below (Pickwell and Sheridan, 1973).

Degree of dissociation

Abnormal retinal correspondence is an adaptation to a squint to prevent the patient being troubled by diplopia in everyday vision. If the conditions of everyday vision are disturbed by dissociating the two eyes in some way, it is likely that normal correspondence will return while the dissociation is present. The more complete the dissociation, the more likely it is that normal correspondence will be present. Applying this factor to some of the tests for correspondence, it will be seen that dissociation is almost total in the after-image test with the eyes closed; with the synoptophore, dissociation is maximal when using simultaneous vision slides which have different pictures for the two eyes, less when fusion slides are used, and least with the Stanworth modification and distance fixation. The striate lenses give least dissociation. The after-image test shows abnormal correspondence in less than 30% of squints, but striate lenses in about 90%.

Retinal areas stimulated

Normal correspondence is most likely to occur with bifoveal images; abnormal correspondence when the fovea of one eye is stimulated simultaneously with a peripheral image in the other eye. The after-image test provides bifoveal or near bifoveal stimulation and therefore will favour normal correspondence. The synoptophore does so when the tubes are set at the true angle of the squint, but setting them at the subjective angle encourages abnormal correspondence. Striate lenses produce foveal – peripheral stimulation and thus strongly favour abnormal correspondence.

Eye used for fixation

Abnormal correspondence is likely when the dominant eye is used for fixation, but normal correspondence is likely to return if the usually squinting eye takes up fixation. Some patients can be persuaded to fix with the eye which usually squints, and under these circumstances the striate lenses may indicate normal correspondence.

Constancy of deviation

If the angle of the squint is variable, abnormal correspondence is less likely to be firmly established. In some cases, the squint may be intermittent, and in these patients normal correspondence will return when the eyes are straight. The same is true of patients with fully accommodative squint when wearing their glasses, in long-standing incomitant squints in the position of no deviation, and in the A and V syndromes in the binocular vision position. Normal correspondence is also likely to occur at the intersections of the visual axes of convergent squints in the physiological diplopia methods of treatment.

Relative illuminance of retinal images

Normal correspondence is more likely to occur if the illuminance of the image in the squinting eye is less than that of the fixing eye. This is the condition when the striate lenses are used with a filter bar, or if the synoptophore tube luminances are unequal.

It is evident that the tests for retinal correspondence form a hierarchy in which normal correspondence is most likely to occur with the after-image tests, and least likely with the striate lenses. The red filter and synoptophore methods occupy intermediate positions. Retinal correspondence may therefore be graded according to whether it is predominantly abnormal, mixed or predominantly normal (see *Table 12.1*).

TABLE 12.1. Clinical classification of anomalous correspondence by depth or grade

Grade of correspondence	*Filter required to produce normal correspondence*	*Tests which give normal correspondence*	*Prognosis*
Predominantly abnormal	Dark	None or only the after-image test	Very poor
Mixed	Medium	After-image and red filter; sometimes with the synoptophore	Fair
Predominantly normal	Light	All tests except striate lenses	Good

Management of abnormal retinal correspondence

In the management of abnormal correspondence, we are concerned mainly with the group of patients showing mixed correspondence. Patients with predominantly normal correspondence may require no treatment other than encouragement of simultaneous macular vision. Those with predominantly abnormal correspondence usually have a bad prognosis: typically these patients have long-standing squint of early onset, and the abnormal correspondence is deeply established. Using striate lenses with a filter bar in predominantly abnormal cases, a very dark filter is required to break down the abnormal correspondence and there is then suppression rather than normal correspondence.

The treatment described may prove successful in those cases of mixed correspondence where all the other factors are hopeful, and may assist early establishment of normal correspondence in those cases where it is already predominantly normal.

Accurate correction of the refractive error is the first essential step. Its effect is two-fold; in accommodative squint the angle is reduced, moving the image in the squinting eye to a more central position where normal correspondence is more likely, and in all squints it ensures that each eye has a sharp retinal image which also aids normal correspondence.

Again, it needs to be emphasized that the abnormal retinal correspondence should not be treated at all if there is little chance of overcoming the deviation. To do so would leave the patient with diplopia. Therefore, in assessing each case, consideration must be given to the possibility of getting rid of the angle. In squints with a deviation over 20^{Δ}, the best approach is to refer for a surgeon's opinion on an operation. It must be remembered, however, that surgery is a 'mechanical solution to a non-mechanical problem' (Dale, 1982), and therefore not the complete answer. Squints between 10^{Δ} and 20^{Δ} may respond to non-surgical methods, and in angles less than 10^{Δ} one has to ask the question about the limits of the accuracy with which surgery can be performed. The question of whether to consider an operation is a matter of professional judgement in each case. Surgeons may be more inclined to recommend it than would other practitioners. The parents also will have a view, and many prefer non-surgical treatment to be tried first. In young patients, the sensory adaptations may disappear or be treated more effectively if the eyes are straightened by an operation first. Where other methods are tried, it is important not to continue with the patient after it is apparent that these methods are not going to be successful, but to seek another opinion while the patient is still young enough for binocular vision to be restored.

Smaller deviations will respond to non-surgical treatment in the form of vergence exercises and other methods. Where this approach is being considered, the first step is to break down the abnormal correspondence. It is very important to be sure that this has been done, before proceeding with the vergence exercises to reduce the angle. The patient must have predominantly normal correspondence before any vergence exercises are carried out.

Amblyopia must also be treated first if the acuity of the squinting eye is not better than 6/24. Occlusion is the best method, since it also weakens the abnormal correspondence.

Other types of treatment for abnormal correspondence should have regard to the five factors which influence the type of correspondence, and which are given above. The aim should be to begin treatment in the conditions which favour normal correspondence, and when this is achieved, move to the less favourable conditions. Consider the factors in the order that they are given above:

(1) *Degree of dissociation* – first try to achieve normal correspondence under maximum dissociation, and then extend this to less and less dissociated conditions. For example, the patient will be able to get normal correspondence with after-images, so that other targets can be introduced and the patient asked to superimpose the after-images on them.
(2) *Retinal areas stimulated* – treatment must be bifoveal or stimulate other normally corresponding areas. Treatment should avoid conditions where the fovea of the dominant eye is presented with an image at the same time as the peripheral area in the other eye which coincides with the angle of squint.
(3) *Eye used for fixation* – if possible, the patient should be taught to fix with the squinting eye as a preliminary to other treatment.
(4) *Constancy of deviation* – try to find conditions in which normal binocular fixation and correspondence is possible, and then extend them to a wider range of circumstances. This is the basis of physiological diplopia methods.
(5) *Relative illuminance of retinal images* – treatment should start from the least inequality of illuminance that will give normal correspondence and move towards more equal illuminance.

The methods of treatment used for abnormal retinal correspondence also help in the treatment of suppression. In squint cases, therefore, it is usually preferable to treat the abnormal correspondence rather than give exercises for suppression alone. As explained earlier in the chapter, any suppression treatment is likely to have the danger of deepening the abnormal correspondence, unless precautions are taken to ensure that there is always stimulation of corresponding points.

There are several approaches to the treatment of abnormal correspondence. The choice of method will depend on the circumstances of the case. Prism therapy methods require less time in supervision and less effort from the patient; physiological diplopia methods can provide integrated binocular vision for one fixation distance, and quite early in treatment; synoptophore methods seem to be more suitable in slightly more difficult cases. The following methods may be considered. They are not necessarily mutually exclusive.

PRISMS

It may be thought that to prescribe full prism relief would provide stimulation of corresponding points and normal correspondence would be re-established. However, a relieving prism in most cases results in the angle of the deviation increasing, sometimes by as much as the original angle of the squint. This phenomenon is known as adaptation to the prism or 'eating up the prisms'. In the majority of cases, prism relief does not work. It has been suggested that a prism adaptation test (Jampolsky, 1971) will help in deciding if the method will work. In a case of convergent squint relieving prism is added before the squinting eye until the cover test shows that a divergent squint is created – a slight overcorrection. This is left in place for some minutes, to see if the adaptation occurs. If the patient adapts only to the excess of prism so that bifoveal fixation is achieved, or if no adaptation occurs, then it is said to be safe to try correction by prism. The overcorrection is recommended. It will be obvious that this prism is going to be a high one and the edge thickness, distortion and appearance are likely to be a problem. Fresnel stick-on prisms can be tried for a few days. They should be placed before the dominant eye, where the slight reduction in acuity may help the amblyopia treatment in the squinting eye. Experience shows that 8^{Δ}–10^{Δ} overcorrection is required, and that even patients who show no prism adaptation at first may do so over a period of a few days. On the whole, treatment by prism relief, even with an overcorrection, does not seem very successful for most patients. Other practitioners have reported this (Mallett, 1979; Dale, 1982).

Vertical prisms in horizontal squint may be more successful. Normal correspondence is easier if the image extends above or below the horizontal: this can be shown by the use of vertical targets. Vertical prism of 6^{Δ}–8^{Δ}, worn base-up and base-down on alternate days, can have the same effect. A clip-on prism has been suggested, but this is cosmetically unacceptable (Mallett, 1979) and it requires a stock of clip-on prisms if one of the right size is to be provided. Fresnel stick-on prisms on the back of the spectacle lens work better.

Mallett (1979) has also advocated the use of adverse prism in breaking down abnormal correspondence: base-in for convergent squint. A prism of 16^{Δ} base-in is recommended as too strong to be overcome by any divergent movement. This produces a rapid breakdown in the abnormal correspondence and it also has a good cosmetic appearance, as the convergent eye looks straighter through the prism.

BASIC SYNOPTOPHORE METHODS

Although many practitioners no longer use a synoptophore, the principles of the methods used with this instrument help our understanding of most other methods. It will also be described for those who wish to use a synoptophore, which can be effective where many other methods are difficult.

The instrument is set at the true objective angle of the squint, and frequent checks must be made at each stage during treatment to ensure that this is maintained so that the instrument presents foveal images to both eyes. This is done by momentarily switching off the tube before the dominant eye in a unilateral squint, or the fixing eye in an alternating squint, and observing the other eye to check that no movement is required for it to take up fixation of the centre of the slide. Alternating illumination should not be used for these checks, as this would allow the build-up to the total angle which is not sustained when both tubes are switched on.

After-images

Some modern synoptophores have a means of providing an after-image in each eye, otherwise the after-images can be created as described above in the section on the investigation of retinal correspondence.

If the patient is asked to observe the after-images against the plane field in the tubes with no slides in the instrument, it is likely that normal correspondence will be observed. Abnormal correspondence under these conditions indicates that it is too deeply established to respond to treatment. Once the patient has observed the cross of the after-images, indicating normal correspondence, a slide can be placed in the tube before one eye, and the patient is asked to see the cross superimposed on the slide picture. A slide with a small central picture before the dominant eye is used first and, when the cross can be seen on it, the slide can be transferred to the other eye. Once normal correspondence is established with one slide, the second slide of a pair can be introduced before the other eye. At first, the patient is asked to concentrate on seeing the crossed after-images, and then gradually to see the two slide pictures superimposed. At any time in this procedure, abnomal correspondence may return and the two slide pictures seen separately. When this occurs, the patient is encouraged to concentrate again on the after-image cross. The after-images are renewed each time they fade.

Alternating exercise

In this method (Chavasse, 1935), the illumination is alternated between the tubes so that each slide is seen in turn. Simultaneous vision slides are used of as small an angular size of picture as the patient can resolve with the amblyopic eye. At first, the rate of alternation is fairly slow – about 1 cycle every 1 or 2 seconds. A time is allowed for the total angle to build up, then the rate of alternation is gradually increased until it becomes physiologically continuous. Hence, the stimulus gradually changes from an alternating monocular one with foveal fixation, to the equivalent of binocular fixation with bifoveal vision. At first, this should give normal correspondence of the foveal images. After a short pause, the patient reports that the images have separated, either because abnormal correspondence has returned or because the angle of the deviation has reverted to the habitual angle. The latter move will be slow, but can be seen either by the practitioner observing the reflections from the cornea of the synoptophore tube lights, or by momentarily switching off the tube before the dominant eye and observing the deviated eye take up fixation. If the decrease in the angle of fixation is not noticed by the practitioner, it may be thought that inharmonious abnormal correspondence has occurred.

Some models of synoptophore have an automated flashing mechanism built into the instrument (Stonebridge, 1951).

Fixation alternation method

The synoptophore tubes are set at an angle slightly greater than the total angle of the squint – about 5^Δ more. This means that in convergent squint there will be crossed diplopia, and the retinal images will be temporal to the fovea and outside the area which may have sensory adaptation. Slides having small simultaneous vision pictures are used. The patient is asked to alternate fixation, looking first at one picture and then at the other, pausing for 1 or 2 seconds at each fixation. As there is abnormal correspondence, the movement will at first appear to be more than separation of 5^Δ, but gradually, or in some cases suddenly, they become seen at their correct separation. The tubes can then be moved so that no movement occurs as the patient alternates fixation. The patient is asked to maintain the images superimposed for as long as possible. When abnormal correspondence recurs, the procedure is repeated.

Macular massage

This expression is used to describe a method in which the tubes are set at the objective angle of the squint to ensure bifoveal images, and one of the tubes is shaken, i.e. moved rapidly back and forwards by a few prism dioptres. This provides a strong stimulation to the fovea of the deviated eye, and encourages normal correspondence with the central image in the undeviated eye.

Kinetic stimulation of corresponding points

The tubes are set at the habitual angle of the deviation and locked into this position. Both tubes can then be moved together, so that the images move across the field while the patient keeps the eyes still. The images then stimulate normally corresponding points across the retina and not just the foveal areas. It is difficult, in this exercise, for the patient to keep the eyes still and not follow the moving target. With a Stanworth synoptophore (see above), a fixation light can be provided across the room and, under the correct levels of illumination of the synoptophore tubes, the patient can maintain fixation as the images move across the retina.

SINGLE MIRROR HAPLOSCOPE

This method provides a good deal of the versatility of the synoptophore, but is much simpler and there is less artificiality, as the patient looks at real objects at an obvious distance rather than images in a tube (Earnshaw, 1962). The general principle of the method is the same as that illustrated in *Figure 12.2* for suppression scotometry. The mirror needs to be firmly mounted so that it can be rotated about a vertical axis to allow adjustment for the angle of the squint. A scale at the base of the pivot will permit measurement of the angular rotation of the mirror if required. It is important that the patient is seated with the eyes an equal distance from each wall, about 1 m, and that the walls are plain so that retinal rivalry is avoided. The practitioner can sit in the corner between the two walls without obscuring the patient's view from either eye. In this position, the eyes can be observed and the cover test performed when required. The targets used can be on card temporarily stuck on the walls in appropriate positions to allow for any vertical deviation if necessary. Most of the methods described for the synoptophore can be carried out in modified form with the single mirror haploscope method. After-images need to be created with a photographic flashgun, but real images can be superimposed on them as required. The fixation alternation method can be carried out by alternating occlusion, and is a method that is particularly appropriate to the single mirror haploscope. Macular massage presents no problems, as the mirror can be rotated back and forth to allow one image to oscillate across the fovea of one eye.

Although this is a very simple type of instrumentation, and works very well under the supervision of the practitioner, experience shows that it presents more difficulties as a home exercise. The idea that it could allow synoptophore-type exercises to be carried out under parent supervision at home seldom seems to work in practice. This is partly because of difficulties in finding a suitably large corner with plain unobstructed walls in very many homes, and partly because of the difficulties in parents being able to observe eye movements well enough to supervise and maintain bifoveal fixation.

FREE SPACE METHODS

Because of the difficulties introduced when patients look through instruments at images rather that at real objects, 'free space' methods of treatment have been developed by various workers in the field (Earnshaw, 1960; Jones, 1965; Gillie and Lindsay, 1969; Hugonnier and Clayette-Hugonnier, 1969; Pickwell, 1971). These methods have been suggested as a follow-up to other treatment at the final stages, but in the case where they are likely to be effective, it is better to use them as the primary form of treatment. Success has been demonstrated in many cases. These seem to be those squints with acuity of 6/24 or better in the amblyopic eye, and with an angle of between 5^{Δ} and 15^{Δ}. For most of these techniques, the starting point is being able to demonstrate a position in front of the eyes where bifoveal fixation can be achieved – the intersection of the visual axes in convergent squint.

After-images in free space

After-images may be used in free space methods as a starting procedure which ensures normal correspondence, or it can be used to supplement other procedures as a check on normal correspondence. The after-images are created by the photographic flashgun masked to provide a line image, or the use of a light bulb as described above. The after-images are best seen against a plain wall initially, to check that the patient localizes them correctly as a cross. They are superimposed on a fixation mark, i.e. a small letter. When this can be done, the patient is asked to touch the letter with the finger tip, and still see the after-images correctly localized. Where the angle of squint cannot be overcome, one eye is occluded.

Physiological diplopia method

This method has been outlined in the previous chapter as a method for the treatment of amblyopia. Where there is abnormal correspondence, the method needs very close supervision so that binocular fixation of the fixation target is always maintained. The practitioner may be able to see by looking at the eyes if they are both fixing or not, and can carry out the cover test at any time that it appears to be in doubt. An intelligent patient can also usually tell when the appearance is correct, but younger children may not be sufficiently reliable in reporting their subjective responses.

As described in the previous chapter, the first step is to find a position where the patient can fix a real object bifoveally. This will be at the intersection of the visual axes in a convergent squint. This position is found by placing a small fixation object at what appears to be the correct distance and carrying out the cover test. The object is moved closer or further away from the eyes until no cover test movement is seen. The patient may have to be encouraged not to overconverge, by explaining that the eyes are looking too close and that one is turned inwards too much. In accommodative squints, a positive spherical addition may be required to inhibit convergence. In those cases where a binocular fixation point can be found, the method may proceed.

A second object is introduced: where abnormal correspondence is present, this second object is placed on the median line and a lot closer to the eyes. By having it closer to the eyes than the fixation object, its image will fall on the temporal retina in each eye. This is to say that in abnormal retinal correspondence cases the nasal retina where sensory adaptations occur is avoided in the early stages until the physiological diplopia has been demonstrated to the patient. A card with differently coloured sides held edgewise against the nose is a useful second object for these early stages. This should be seen in crossed physiological diplopia; the patient should see the fixation object singly with the coloured patch from the right of the card in the left periphery of vision, and the coloured patch from the left of the card seen in the right periphery.

The fixation object and card are shown in *Figure 8.7,* which illustrates also a length of string which can be introduced at a later stage. At this stage, rather than a continuous string it is better to use a third object further away from the fixation but of the same nature. Coloured pencils are suitable, or thin rods or needles mounted in plasticine to stand vertically on a table. The third object should be about 15 cm beyond the first and also on the median line. The patient is encouraged to see this object in uncrossed physiological diplopia, but to maintain fixation on the first object. The patient is then taught to maintain physiological diplopia of the more distant object while it is moved slowly towards the fixation object. If physiological diplopia is lost or the practitioner sees that the eyes have converged, the more distant object is temporarily removed and fixation re-established.

If the patient sees both diplopic images on the same side – paradoxical diplopia – the fixation object is no longer at the intersection of the axes, and proper fixation needs to be re-established. A small vertical after-image on the fovea may assist as a subjective check on central fixation. The fixation object can also be changed for a small light, and this allows the use of striate lenses as a check on retinal correspondence.

With practice and encouragement, the patient should be able to achieve steady fixation of the first object and physiological diplopia of the more distant one, while the latter is moved from its initial position to a position 4 or 5 cm from the fixation. The methods described in Chapter 8 can then proceed as an extension of this exercise.

It is very important not to move the fixation object from its best position until normal correspondence is well established. In the very early stages of treatment, it is better to concentrate on establishing binocular fixation with physiological diplopia at one distance only, and develop this with some of the suppression exercises described in Chapter 8 or earlier in this chapter: wire reading, bar reading, etc. This is to concentrate on the sensory aspects of the squint rather than the actual motor deviation. Indeed, in some cases, once the sensory problems are sorted out, it is found that the deviation is present neither at near nor distance vision, but this spontaneous recovery for the deviation does not necessarily occur. It will then be necessary to give vergence exercises.

Vergence exercises

When the sensory adaptations to the squint have been treated and a level of acuity of 6/12 or better has been established, attention should be given to the motor deviation by vergence exercises. It is very important that this is not done too early or there will be a danger of abnormal retinal correspondence returning. Most of the prism vergence exercises described in Chapter 8 can be considered at this stage. It must be remembered, however, that treatment will begin at the angle of the squint and not the orthophoria position.

As mentioned above, it is very unlikely that angles of squint greater than 20^{Δ} will respond to non-surgical treatment alone, and in cases of 15^{Δ}–20^{Δ}, all other factors need to be favourable before attempting orthoptic treatment.

References

BAGOLINA, I. (1971). Anomalous binocular vision and suppression in strabismic patients. *Transactions of the International Congress of the British Optical Association*, pp. 298–307

CHAVASSE, B. (1935). Test for secondary correspondence in squint. *Transactions of the Ophthalmological Society of the United Kingdom*, **55**, 482–498

DALE, R. T. (1982). *Fundamentals of Ocular Motility and Strabismus*. Grune & Stratton, New York

EARNSHAW, J. R. (1960). The use of knitting needles in the treatment of strabismus. *Optician*, **139**, 465–466.

EARNSHAW, J. R. (1962). The single mirror haploscope. *Transactions of the International Congress of the British Optical Association*, pp. 673–674

GILLIE, J. C. and LINDSAY, M. A. (1969). *Orthoptics: A Discussion of Binocular Anomalies*. Hatton Press, London

HUGONNIER, R. and CLAYETTE-HUGONNIER, S. (1969). *Strabismus, Heterophoria, Ocular Motor Paralysis* (translated and edited by S, Verroneau-Troutman). Mosby, St. Louis

JAMPOLSKY, A. (1971). A simplified approach to strabismus diagnosis, in *Symposium of Strabismus*. Mosby, St. Louis, pp. 3–4

JONES, B. A. (1965). Orthoptic handling of fusion vergences. *American Orthoptic Journal*, **15**, 21–29

MALLETT, R. F. (1979). The use of prisms in the treatment of concomitant strabismus. *The Ophthalmic Optician*, **19**, 793–798

PICKWELL, L. D. (1971). Simple methods in everyday orthoptics. *Optician*, **161**(4177), 10–12

PICKWELL, L. D. and SHERIDAN, M. (1973) The management of ARC. *The Ophthalmic Optician*, **13**(11), 588–592

STANWORTH, A. (1958). Modified major amblyoscope. *British Journal of Ophthalmology*, **42**, 270–287

STONEBRIDGE, E. H. (1951). The Stonebridge electronic alternator. *Optician*, **121**(3140), 555–557, 561

13

Microtropia

Microsquint, or microtropia (Lang, 1966), may be found as an apparently primary condition, or it may be present as a residual deviation after the treatment of a larger squint. It has been suggested that it has inherited characteristics (Burian and von Noorden, 1974): anisometropia is often a major factor, and a foveal scotoma results from the confusion of the blurred image with the sharp one in the other eye. It appears to develop before the age of 3 years, but it may break down into a larger angle squint and give the impression that a squint has come on in later childhood. It is usually an eso-deviation.

Clinical characteristics

The terminology surrounding very small angle squints has been very confused, but microsquint is now recognized as having the following characteristics in very many cases:

(1) *Small angle*. The microsquint is less than 6^{Δ} in angle. The deviation may not show on the cover test; not because it is too small, but because it is a fully adapted squint (see below). Sometimes a small deviation is manifest.

(2) *Anisometropia*. There is usually a difference between the refractive errors in the two eyes of more than 1.50 D. Occasionally, microsquint will be found in patients with equal refractive errors.

(3) *Amblyopia*. There is reduced acuity in one eye, and as the deviation may not be apparent on the cover test, the amblyopia may be the first indication of the microsquint. Unually the acuity is only reduced one or two lines to 6/9 or 6/12 (20/30 or 20/40).

(4) *Eccentric fixation*. Central fixation is always lost in microsquint. There is a suppression scotoma and often an absolute scotoma in the foveal area of the amblyopic eye. The angle of the eccentricity of the fixation is usually the same as the angle of the squint, and this is the reason why the eye does not move on the cover test: the area of the retina on which the image falls in binocular vision is the same as the eccentrically fixing area (the area used for fixation when the other eye is covered). Occasionally, in microsquint, the degree of eccentric fixation is less than the angle of the squint, and in these cases a very small cover test movement may be seen.

(5) *Abnormal correspondence.* Harmonious abnormal correspondence is present in microsquint. Therefore, it will be seen that in most cases there will be identity of the retinal area on which the image falls in the patient's habitual vision with both the area used for fixation and the anomalously corresponding area. This has been referred to as microsquint with identity, but most microsquint is of this type; that is, the squint is fully adapted.

(6) *Peripheral fusion.* The eyes in microsquint seem to be held in the nearly straight position of the small angle by the fusional impulses provided by peripheral vision. There may be amplitude of fusion which can be measured in the same way as prism vergences.

(7) *Monofixational syndrome.* In many cases of microsquint, the angle of the deviation may increase on the alternating cover test or even if one eye is covered for a slightly longer time than normal for the cover test. When the cover is removed from both the eyes, the eye which was last covered will be seen to return to the microsquint position. There is the appearance of esophoria in spite of the microsquint. It is as if a heterophoric movement is superimposed on the squint. The apparent heterophoria may be larger and more obvious than the microsquint, which may not show at all on the cover test. A microsquint showing the superimposed esophoria movement is known as the monofixational syndrome or monofixational heterophoria (Parks and Eustis, 1961; Parks, 1969).

(8) *Stereopsis.* A low grade of stereopsis has been reported in microsquint (Okuda, Apt and Wanter, 1977), but this has not been confirmed using standard clinical tests (Pickwell and Jenkins, 1978).

Investigation and diagnosis

The investigation and diagnosis of microsquint follow a full routine examination, but the following aspects are particularly useful in the detection of this condition.

ACUITY

The presence of amblyopia in one eye is usually the first clue that microsquint may be found. The amblyopic eye usually shows the crowding phenomenon referred to in Chapter 11; that is, single letter acuity is better than line acuity. The foveal scotoma may also result in the patient missing out letters when reading lines of Snellen letters, or he or she may read the line more easily backwards (see *Figure 11.1*).

FIXATION

The presence of eccentric fixation should be checked with the ophthalmoscopic method and by one other means. The eccentric fixation may be seen by the very small difference between the position of the corneal reflection of a monocularly fixed light in each eye in turn (see Chapter 11 for the investigation of eccentric fixation).

COVER TEST

As explained above, the microsquint is unlikely to be detected as a strabismic movement with the cover test. The presence of the monofixational syndrome may be seen as an apparent heterophoria movement when the cover is removed, and this could result in the microsquint being missed.

FOUR PRISM DIOPTRE TEST

In this test (Irvine, 1948), if a 4^{Δ} base-out prism is placed before the dominant eye, the image will be moved across the retina and the eye will move inwards to take up fixation. Because of Hering's law of equal eye movements, the other eye will move laterally in the same direction. This versional movement of both eyes can be seen by the practitioner rather than a convergent movement in a subject with normal binocular vision. When the prism is removed, there will be a recovery movement of both eyes laterally and in the same direction. If the prism is placed before the amblyopic eye, the image will move across the retina within the suppression area, and there will be no movement of either eye. In cases where there is amblyopia in one and and no movement on the normal cover test, the above responses to the four prism dioptre tests confirms a microsquint.

STRIATE LENS TEST

If a vertical streak is produced by placing a striate lens before the amblyopic eye, the patient will report that the streak passes through the spot of light, or is in line with it, there being a central gap caused by the suppression scotoma. This indicates harmonious abnormal correspondence.

AMSLER CHARTS

The scotoma may show on the Amsler charts or as a disturbance of a page of print (see the section on the investigation of eccentric fixation in Chapter 11).

Management

Microsquint is a fully adapted squint and does not give rise to symptoms unless other conditions have been superimposed. Management consists, initially, of correcting the refractive error. This is particularly important if the patient is under 5 years of age and has anisometropia. Orthoptic treatment for the microsquint is very seldom successful, and is not worth trying in patients over the age of 4 or 5 years. Under this age, all the problems of giving treatment for eccentric fixation to a very young child reduce the chances of success considerably. In most cases, therefore, correction of the refractive error is the only profitable action.

If the microsquint has broken down into a larger deviation, or if monofixational heterophoria is decompensated and giving rise to symptoms, treatment for these conditions may be appropriate to restore the microsquint to its compensated and fully adapted state. The treatment in such cases will consist of that described in the earlier chapters for esophoria and esotropia – suppression and vergence exercises.

References

BURIAN, H. M. and VON NOORDEN, G. K. (1974). *Binocular Vision and Ocular Motility*. Mosby, St. Louis, p. 295

IRVINE, S. R. (1948). Amblyopia ex anopsia. *Transactions of the American Ophthalmological Society*, **46,** 527

LANG, J. (1966). Evaluation in small angle strabismus or microtropia, in *International Strabismus Symposium* (Ed. A. Arruga). University of Giessen, Basel, p. 219

OKUDA, F. C., APT, A. and WANTER, B. S. (1977). Evaluation of the random dot stereogram tests. *American Orthoptic Journal*, **28,** 124–130

PARKS, M. M. (1969). The monofixational syndrome. *Transactions of the American Ophthalmological Society*, **67,** 609

PARKS, M. M. and EUSTIS, A. J. (1961). Monofixational phoria. *American Orthoptic Journal*, **11,** 38

PICKWELL, L. D. and JENKINS, T. C. A. (1978). Using the Titmus stereotest. *Optician*, **175,** 17, 19

14

Examination of young children

Objectives

In examining the eyes and vision of pre-school age children under the age of 5 years, our approach and method have to be modified from the routine appropriate to older children and adults. It is likely that there will be much less co-operation on the part of the very young patient so we need to use quick simple tests that can be applied for the short time we can count on the patient's attention. Precise measurements may not always be possible, and we have to look for significant departures from normal. That is to say, there is much more of a screening element in the investigation of pre-school children.

A young child cannot give subjective symptoms and we have to rely on the observation and impressions of the parent. The family history will be very important. Children whose parents or whose brothers or sisters have squint or amblyopia are very much more likely to develop these conditions.

Active pathology

As with all patients, anomalies of binocular vision in children may be a sign of active pathology. The first responsibility of the practitioner is to investigate this possibility. Where there is any doubt, the patient will need to be referred for medical investigation before proceeding. The following points are particularly stressed:

(1) *Check for incomitancy* – this is usually possible where there is a large deviation by holding the child's head still and attracting the attention so that the eyes turn into the tertiary positions of gaze
(2) *Note the palpebral openings* – the two lid openings should be equal and symmetrical. Any inequality in a squinting child may indicate a growth of extra tissue in the orbit. This would push the eye forward and disturb the eye movements. It could be caused by a dermoid cyst, sarcoma of the muscles or glioma of the optic nerve.
(3) *Ophthalmoscopy* – an attempt should be made to look at the media and fundus, but look at the colour of the fundus reflex, even if a full ophthalmoscopic examination is not possible. This may be done with an

ophthalmoscope, or with a retinoscope moved around so that all areas of the fundus are checked: the retinoscope gives a narrow concentrated beam of light, and can be used from a greater distance, which may more readily be tolerated by the patient. White areas of the fundus are a sign of retinoblastoma, and a squint may be the first sign of this condition, which usually begins before the age of 4 years.

It must be remembered that there are methods of investigation which are available in most hospitals, but are seldom possible in outside practices. It is essential that very young patients have the benefit of these hospital facilities where there is the slightest doubt.

Development of vision

In order to be able to assess the eyes and the vision of infants, it is important that we should have some idea of how vision normally develops from birth through infancy and childhood to adult vision. Although a lot more is now known about this, there are still many gaps in our knowledge. Normal vision requires a good optical system with a focused image and good resolution. Optical resolution has also to be matched with a neural receptor system of good resolution and a neural image processing ability leading to psychological perception. The perceptive level itself is very dependent on previous visual and other sensory experience. Obviously this sensory experience cannot be present at birth. As experience grows, reflexes are reinforced and associations between different sensory input and experiences are formed. For example, it is clear that very early in life an infant learns to recognize the mother's face and the meaning of different facial expressions. All visual functions are built as they are reinforced by experience acting on the anatomical and physiological systems which, although not complete at birth, mature early in life and allow the full potential of the visual system to develop. This is true for fixation, acuity, sensory fusion, motor fusion and stereopsis.

Fixation

The ability to fix is not present at birth but normally develops as the myelination of the nerve fibres is completed in the first 2 or 3 weeks. Before then the eyes are unstable in their position which is determined at this stage mainly by the vestibular reflexes. The fixation reflex requires reinforcement by active vision if it is to develop normally. If the system is faulty in some way, this may prevent normal development of central fixation and therefore normal acuity. Each eye requires a central and sharply focused image and a fully developed neural system in order that fixation may become stable and acuity develop to the adult level of 6/5. Normally, the retina and the rest of the visual neural system are adequately developed soon after birth. The infant learns to turn the eyes to obtain a central foveal image in both eyes during the first month of life. This fixation reflex is not firmly established until later and if anything impedes it during the first 2 or 3 months of life, central fixation can easily be lost. This period of 2 or 3 months when development is taking place is known as the critical period so far as fixation is concerned. The critical period for acuity development is 2 or 3 years (see below). It is followed by a further period during which the system can easily break down. This is called the plastic period and central fixation can still be lost up to the age of 3 years if anything disturbs the system.

Occasionally there are abnormalities in the foveal nervous system which are present from birth, but these account for only a very small number of eyes with fixation failure. Most loss of fixation arises from the lack of a central image in a squinting eye or occasionally from a very blurred image. If either of these is present during the critical period there will be a failure of normal fixation and acuity to develop, and unless treatment is given before the end of the plastic period, it is very unlikely that central fixation can ever be achieved. The longer the squint or the blurred vision is left untreated, the less chance there is of ever getting central fixation with full acuity. This obviously emphasizes the need for early detection and treatment. It has also been shown that if an eye is occluded for a long time for any reason during the critical period, this too will impede the acuity development, deprivation amblyopia. If the occlusion occurs before the age of several months, central fixation will also be lost.

The critical period varies for each of the visual functions. Binocular integration has a different but largely overlapping time scale. Stereopsis seems to develop later (Vital-Durand, 1987).

Sensory fusion

Binocular vision is developed at about the same rate as the fixation reflex, and the same considerations apply to it. The anatomical and physiological potential is present at birth, and it requires regular reinforcement to become established. Cortical cells require an input from both eyes if they are to become the 'binocularly driven' cells of the normal adult system. This must occur during the critical period. A squint or occlusion of one eye will prevent this bi-foveal stimulation, and if not checked during the critical period, binocular vision may never be possible as the binocularly driven cells will not develop but become monocular cells. Obviously the 'infantile esotropia syndrome' with its onset under the age of one year needs early referral. If such patients are not seen until they are over a year old, it is very unlikely that anything other than a cosmetic operation will help. Indeed, the prognosis for achieving binocular vision in infantile esotropia is never very good.

Motor fusion

The ability of the two eyes to make vergence movements in order to obtain a foveal image in both also develops with the fixation reflex. It is demonstrated when the child changes fixation distance and makes a fusional vergence movement. It can also be demonstrated by placing a 10 dioptre prism base-out before one eye. If there is normal motor fusion, a convergent movement will be seen, and a divergent movement as the prism is removed. Motor fusion is reinforced during the critical period by developments in the motor components of the visual system which are comparable with those of the sensory fusion system in the cortex.

It is likely that the pursuit reflex is also developed concurrently so that the eyes can follow a moving object and maintain a foveal image of it. In infantile esotropia there is usually crossed fixation so that fixation occurs with the right eye for objects in the left field and with the left eye for objects in the right of the field. Under these circumstances, the pursuit reflex may develop normally in each eye for half the field. In the other half, the eye may not follow correctly if the other eye is covered. This will give the appearance of a lateral rectus palsy. (As the crossed fixation is a form of alternating squint, it usually allows the development of good acuity.)

Versions, vergences and accommodation

Versional movements develop with the fixation, but vergence reflexes are not present until about 6 months of age. Both need reinforcing by unimpeded use and can easily breakdown or fail to be established if there is a problem.

The evidence on accommodation is more conflicting due to the difficulty of measurement. It is reasonable to suppose that accommodative reflexes require sufficient acuity to detect the blur which is the principal stimulus. However, Haynes, White and Held (1965) using dynamic retinoscopy found evidence to suggest that changes in accommodation can be detected as early as 4 months.

Acuity

The rate at which acuity develops in human infants depends on how it is defined and on how it is investigated. Using the objective assessment of the visually evoked response (VER), it appears that the infant's ability to resolve patterns improves from a level equivalent to less than 6/60 soon after birth to the equivalent of 6/5 during the first 6 months of life. The 'preferential looking' method relies on observing whether the infant turns the head and eyes to look at a grating rather than a grey patch of equal size and luminance. If no preference is shown for the grating, it is assumed that it cannot be resolved. This method indicates that 6/5 acuity is not reached until after one year of age. Physiological optico-kinetic nystagmus (OKN) in response to a moving grating shows a similar rate of acuity development. Obviously a Snellen type acuity measurement cannot be made until the child is older even if specially designed tests are used; e.g. Sheridan-Gardner (STYCAR) test, Ffookes symbols or tumbling Es. However, these are the tests most readily available in optometric practice. They suggest that 6/5 acuity is not achieved until over the age of 3 years. All these Snellen type tests however involve an element of form perception. At the simplest, the child must be able to recognize the difference between a square, a circle or a triangle. Form perception is developed later than system resolution, so that Snellen type measurements are a more advanced form of vision.

Refractive error

The refractive error during the first year of life is very variable in most infants. At birth it is of the order of +2.00 DS (SD = 2.00 DS). It is approximately +2.50 DS in about 50% of infants. There is hyperopic astigmatism in 29% and myopia in 23% (Cook and Glasscock, 1951). In many infants, high degrees of astigmatism are observed during the first year, but this is variable and disappears before the end of the first year.

Over one year of age, hyperopia over +4.00 DS can be of significance in the cause of accommodative squint. At the age of 3 years, refractive error over +2.50 DS indicates the need for investigation of binocular vision at regular intervals. Anisometropia of more than 1.00 D or astigmatism over 1.00 D at any age over one year indicates the need for a correction to be considered. Normal acuity development requires a good and equally sharp image in both eyes.

Stereopsis

Stereopsis is not demonstrated until after the age of 3 years. Romano, Romano and Puklin (1976) using the Titmus test, found that at first the stereo-acuity is low,

3000″. At 5 years it had improved to 140″, and did not reach a normal adult value of 40″ until the age of 9 years. It appears to be a little better with the TNO test. After the age of 3, the demonstration of stereopsis establishes the presence of binocular vision with good acuities and compensated heterophoria.

Examination

During the examination the child should sit on the mother's knee, where he or she will feel more secure in otherwise strange surroundings. The mother may be able to help in eliciting the child's attention when required, or in steadying the head. Give time for the patient to get used to the situation while you are taking the history and symptoms from the mother. Try to relate to the child in a friendly way at appropriate moments before carrying out any 'tests'. Where possible, tests are presented as games to be played. A third adult in the room may be of help in holding test cards and fixation targets for distance vision. Do not darken the room unless absolutely necessary. It is better to wear informal clothing, and to avoid clinical white coats, etc.

Equipment

Some extra equipment may be useful, depending on the exact age of the patient. Small attractive toys to hold attention for fixation are necessary, and picture books may be useful. Suitable acuity tests such as the Sheridan–Gardiner test, Ffooks symbols, picture charts or 'E' cards need to be available. Lens racks are designed

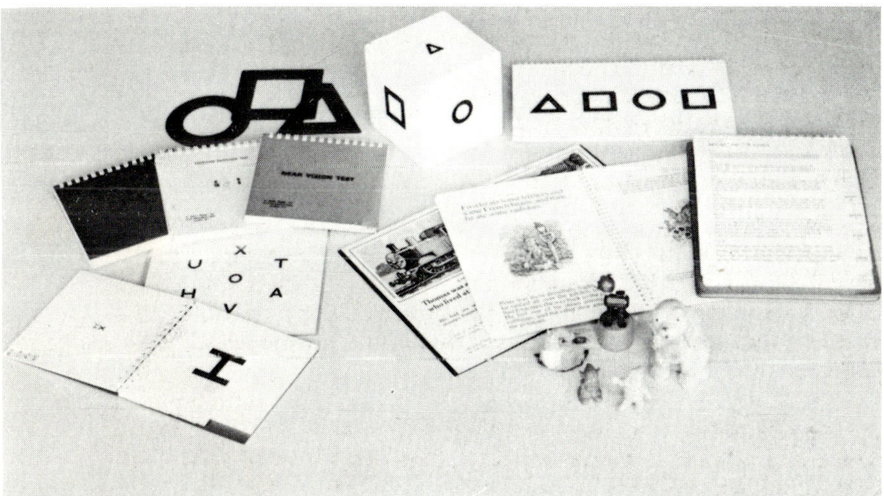

Figure 14.1. Acuity tests for young children. Ffooks tests (top) – the book of distance vision charts is shown on the right, a cube with Ffooks symbols is in the centre, and the cut-out shapes to help the child identify the symbols seen is on the left. Sheridan–Gardiner test (left) – the books of letters are shown, together with the identification card. Examples of near-vision test cards for children include the Maclure test types which are graded for type size and the age of the patient (right). Also shown (bottom right) are examples of toys suitable for fixation targets for young children – the largest toy will also squeak to aid attracting attention

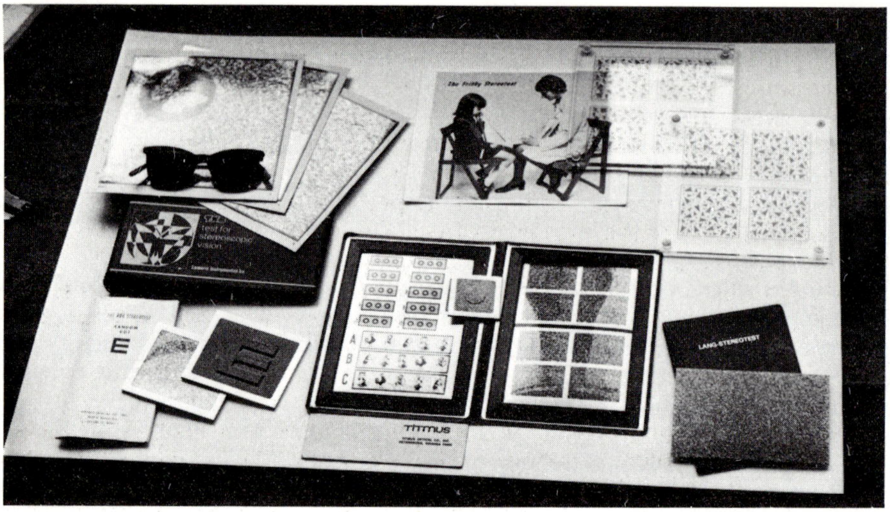

Figure 14.2. Stereoscopic tests: TNO test (top left); Frisby test (top right); Stereo random dot E test (bottom left); Titmus random dot test (centre); Lang test (bottom right)

for use with children who are too young to wear a trial frame, and a headband-supported trial frame is sometimes useful. Often single trial lenses can be hand held before the eye as the most effective method. Refractor heads and phoroptors are not appropriate to young children. A stereotest should be available. The TNO test can be used on quite young patients, as can the Wirt fly test (see *Figures 14.1* and *14.2*).

Methods

As explained above, the normal routine examination is not appropriate to children under the age of 5 years. We therefore need to decide exactly what we want to know as a minimum, and the quickest way to arrive at an answer. If a squint is suspected, the priorities are to ask the following questions:

(1) Is binocular vision present?
(2) Are there any signs of a squint?
(3) Is the unaided vision the same in the two eyes?
(4) Is the refractive error normal or nearly normal for the age?
(5) Is the corrected acuity normal for the age?

It may not be possible to answer all these questions for every child. With others, much more can be done in addition. A lot will depend on the level of co-operation of the young patient. Great patience and more than one visit may be required. The following procedures are suggested in answering the above questions.

BINOCULAR VISION

The first step is to try to discover if there is binocular vision, and this may be indicated in children over 6 months by attracting the child's attention and placing a prism base out of 10^{Δ} or 20^{Δ} before one eye and noting any fusional movement that

LTC

occurs to compensate for the prism. A convergent movement of the eye shows that binocular vision is present; a versional movement suggests that the other eye is not fixing, and the prism should be tried before this eye. If no movement is seen, it suggests that binocular vision is doubtful.

Even patients as young as $2\frac{1}{2}$ years will sometimes co-operate enough to respond to the Wirt fly test by slight repulsion if the fly is seen in three dimensions. With children over 3 years, better stereopsis may be present. If asked to nip the wing, the fingers should be clear of the page by 5–10 cm. The TNO test will also show readily if binocular vision is present in quite young patients.

Often, these tests are enough in themselves to show that there is no serious reason for suspecting a squint. The tests should be repeated every 3–6 months.

COVER TEST

It is usually possible to perform the cover test with near fixation on most infants of 6 months or over, if patience is exercised and the practitioner takes advantage of the moments when the child is fixing. The palm of the hand is used for occlusion rather than any other 'occluder' which distracts attention. The objective should be to reveal any strabismic movements. Sometimes, it is obvious that the patient objects to one eye being covered but not the other, suggesting a difference in acuity.

The deviation which is present from a very early age is the 'infantile esotropia syndrome' or congenital convergent squint. It usually has a large angle – over 40^{Δ} – which is the same for distance and near fixation. There is often a higher degree of hyperopia than normal for the age and the deviation may be partially accommodative. There is usually crossed alternating fixation; that is, the right eye tends to fix objects in the left part of the visual field, and the left eye fixes in the right field. The change of fixation can be seen if the patient can be persuaded to follow a target moved across the horizontal. It seems that about half the patients have amblyopia with eccentric fixation (Dale, 1982). There may be latent nystagmus (see Chapter 17), and sometimes alternating sursumduction (see Chapter 7, p. 69).

Another infantile anomaly is the 'nystagmus compensation (or blocking) syndrome' (von Noorden, 1976). In this condition, the convergent squint seems to be adopted in order to lessen nystagmoid movements which are reduced on convergence of the eyes. The patient's head is usually turned away from the side of the fixing eye so as to produce further convergence of this eye, and there may be the appearance of a lateral rectus palsy (see Chapter 16).

Neither of these conditions can be treated by refractive or orthoptic means alone, and a surgeon's opinion should be taken as soon as possible.

MOTILITY TEST

In the case of a very young patient, this test may be possible using small toys as fixation if the patient does not look at a pentorch. If a squint is suspected, it is important to know if possible whether it is comitant.

UNCORRECTED VISION

Uncorrected vision and acuity with any spectacle correction can be measured with appropriate children's tests. Children who cannot easily name letters can be asked to point to the same letter as the one in the distance if a card is provided with a selection of letters. This is the basis of the Sheridan–Gardiner test (see *Figure 14.1*).

For younger children, letter designs may be too complicated, and the more simple test which asks them to discriminate between a circle, a triangle and a square may be better. The Ffooks test is of this design, but even with this it must not be assumed that a child can necessarily tell the difference between these shapes, and it may be necessary to teach the patient to do so first. Again, it may be more appropriate to ask the patient to point to cut-out shapes held close enough to touch rather than to ask the patient to name the shapes. Alternatively, the patient can be asked to draw the letter or the shape in the air with a finger.

OPHTHALMOSCOPY

As some squint in children under the age of 5 may be due to a pathological cause, it is very important to make a valid attempt at ophthalmoscopy. Usually, in children, the pupil is large and the media clear, which helps in seeing the fundus. The indirect method may be more appropriate to get an overall view of the fundus quickly.

REFRACTION

Initially, we need to discover if there is any significant refractive error, rather than to measure the exact degree: is there more hyperopia than normal for the age, astigmatism greater than 1 D, anisometropia more than 2 D, or is there myopia? Any of these indicate a need for further investigation, but otherwise the patient can be checked again in 6 months.

The refraction will need to be carried out objectively. Hold a single trial case sphere before one eye, and observe the type of movement with the retinoscope. The power of the sphere will be the average refraction for the age, plus 1 DS, plus the 'working distance' lens; for example, in a patient of 2 years, $+3.75 + 1.00 + 2.00 = +6.75$ DS (say +7.00 DS). It is better to work at a distance of half a metre for very young patients. A 'with' movement indicates that more hyperopia is present. Any significant astigmatism can be seen. An 'against' movement may indicate less hyperopia or that the patient is accommodating. A cycloplegic refraction can follow at a second visit of the patient. The corrected acuity can also be measured. During the cycloplegic examination, the patient can be encouraged to fix the retinoscope light.

In cases where the co-operation of the patient is poor, it may be useful to attempt the more simple 'Bruckner test' first (Griffin and Cotter, 1986). The ophthalmoscope which has a fairly divergent beam is held at about 40 cm from the child's eyes so that the fundus reflex can be seen in both eyes at the same time. The two reflexes are compared. Any obvious differences in the distribution of the light indicate anisometropia. Other observations can be made at the same time: pupil reflexes; the positions of the corneal reflections may indicate a deviation; opacities in the media; disturbances in iris pattern; or white patches on the fundus.

A fairly reliable assessment of the refractive state can also be obtained by photo-refraction. This is a system by which the refractive error can be calculated from the apparent size of the fundus light patch in the pupil in two photographs taken with the camera focused at two levels. A computerized system is available which records the reflex sizes from a video-camera and almost instantly calculates the refraction. This system is most useful in situations where a lot of infants are seen.

Management

First, the question of a referral for medical investigation should be considered, and this is essential if there is any doubt about the presence of pathology. It should also be recommended where it is clear that the circumstances would not allow a reasonable prognosis to refractive and orthoptic treatment. If the patient is going to require medical attention, the sooner the referral the better. Care should be taken not to delay other treatment when it is clear that the condition will not respond to the methods available.

Patients in this age group are often too young to co-operate with any form of orthoptic exercises. Refractive error should be corrected if possible, and any amblyopia treated by total occlusion. The occluder is worn on the dominant eye for 3 days, and then changed to the other eye for 1 day to allow development of acuity in the dominant eye. Occlusion may be required for several months, so that the alternation of the occluder is important in these very young cases. Such cases should be kept under close supervision, and the patient needs to be seen at frequent intervals to check progress and be reassessed, so that orthoptic exercises can begin as soon as the patient is old enough to co-operate.

Modern methods of acuity assessment in very young children suggest that vision develops at a much earlier age than previously believed. This emphasizes the need for examination as early as possible, so that measures can be taken to prevent the failure of the development of acuity which results in amblyopia and may be difficult to treat later. Children whose parents (or other close relative) have amblyopia or squint are ten times more likely to have amblyopia than other children. It is therefore particularly important that these children should be seen as early in life as possible, and that young adult patients with amblyopia should be advised that their children's eyes need examining.

The general principles of squint management are described in Chapter 15.

References

COOK, R. C. and GLASSCOCK, R. E. (1951). Refractive and ocular findings in the newborn. *American Journal of Optometry*, **34,** 1407–1413

DALE, R. T. (1982). *Fundamentals of Ocular Motility and Strabismus.* Grune & Stratton, New York, pp. 201–202

GRIFFIN, J. R. and COTTER, S. A. (1986). Evaluation of clinical usefulness of the Bruckner test. *American Journal of Optometry,* **63**(12), 957–961

HAYNES, H. M., WHITE, B. L. and HELD, R. (1965). Visual accommodation in human infants. *Science,* **148,** 582

NOORDEN, G. K. VON (1976). The hystagmus compensation (blocking) syndrome. *American Journal of Ophthalmology,* **82,** 283–290

ROMANO, P. E., ROMANO, J. A. and PUKLIN, J. E. (1976). The development of normal binocular single vision in childhood. *Orthoptics; Past, Present and Future,* edited by S. Moore, J. Mein and L. Stockbridge. pp. 11–160. Stratton Corporation, New York

VITAL-DURAND, F. (1987). The neural basis of deprivation amblyopia in the monkey. *Transactions of the 6th International Orthoptic Congress:* British Orthoptic Society, London

15 Evaluation and management of squint

Following the initial examination of a patient with squint, an evaluation of all the information available needs to be carried out in order to decide the management of each patient. Many squints need referral for medical investigation and possible surgery. Others are entirely within the province of optometric management.

Many patients are adults and of an age when it is not possible to restore binocular vision. Those with a recent onset and distressing symptoms obviously need medical investigation. Most of the other adult squinters have come to terms with the anomaly and require spectacles for their refractive problems only. Many children, however, respond to optometric treatment. Obviously there is a need to define the types of squint likely to be found in optometric practice, and understand the best form of approach to each. It is in nobody's interest to hold on to a patient who would be better referred. Indeed, to keep a patient on ineffective treatment too long can reduce the chance of success by other methods. Equally, if the treatment required is optometric, it should receive optometric attention.

Time of onset

The first critical question is the time of onset of the squint. It can be difficult to be sure of this as parents are not always reliable in their information. Photographs taken in the first year may help. The important thing to establish is whether the deviation was present during the first year of life.

Squints with an onset before one year

The investigation by full routine examination should show the type of squint present. Squints with an age of onset before one year are now classified as being the infantile esotropia syndrome (or congenital squint). They may be further subdivided as 'essential infantile esotropia', nystagmus blocking syndrome, or may be a sixth nerve palsy. (See Chapter 14 in the cover test description.) None of these squints will respond to optometric treatment regardless of the age at which the patient is seen. When these types of squint are found in young children, they should be referred for a surgeon's opinion. If the patient is over the age of 6 or 7, it is unlikely that anything other than a cosmetic improvement will result. Sometimes an accommodative squint occurs under the age of a year. The earlier treatment begins with these patients, the better the chances of success (for management, see below).

Divergent squint which is present from birth is usually associated with some sort of neurological condition. It is very unusual to see a congenital exotropia in an otherwise normal infant (Moore and Cohen, 1985). These squints do not respond to optometric treatment and should be referred for medical advice.

Squints with an onset after one year

REFRACTIVE

In some squints, the refractive error is part of the cause of the deviation and therefore the refractive correction is a major part of the treatment. Refractive (or optometric) squints may be considered under three headings:

(1) *Fully accommodative:* in some squints, the deviation is secondary to the presence of hyperopia. There is usually a degree of hyperopia over +3.00 DS which requires a young patient to accommodate to obtain clear vision for distance and to accommodate excessively for near vision. Because of the relationship between accommodation and convergence, this abnormal accommodation stimulates excessive convergence which, in some young patients, is sufficient to cause a squint. The AC/A ratio in accommodative squint may be normal.

In the fully accommodative squint, correction of the hyperopia relieves the accommodation and eliminates the deviation. It is important that treatment begins at as early an age as possible. The management of this type of squint therefore consists of prescribing the full cycloplegic refractive findings for constant wear. The effect on the binocular vision should be checked in 3 or 4 weeks. Any suppression still present should be treated by simultaneous vision exercises with a Holmes stereoscope, by bar reading or by physiological diplopia appreciation methods (see Chapter 8).

In children, it is expected that binocular vision can be restored and that there will be an improvement in the acuity of the amblyopic eye. If the starting acuity is less than 6/12, a period of direct occlusion of the non-squinting eye may assist in patients under the age of 7 years.

(2) *Partially accommodative:* in some squints, the deviation is reduced by the hyperopic correction to a small residual angle. The management of this type of squint depends on the size of the residual angle, the depth of the sensory adaptations, the age of the patient, and level of co-operation of the patient and parents. It is a matter of clinical judgement whether to treat by optometric methods or refer for a surgeon's opinion. Where the residual angle is small, the patient young with an onset of the squint in the last few years, and the level of co-operation is likely to be good, these cases will respond to orthoptic treatment.

Again a full cycloplegic refractive correction for constant wear is prescribed. The physiological diplopia methods can be successful in these cases. This is particularly true if a point of binocular fixation can be found in front of the eyes where the visual axes cross, if an object is placed at this point and fixation checked with the cover test. It may be possible that a second object placed closer to eyes can be appreciated in crossed physiological diplopia. Or if this produces an increase in the angle of the squint, an object placed further from the eyes than the fixation object may be appreciated in uncrossed physiological diplopia, while fixation is maintained. Either of these conditions represents a limited form of binocular vision at this particular fixation distance. It is a starting point from which to overcome suppression by moving the second object closer to the first while maintaining binocular fixation of the first object and the appreciation of the physiological diplopia. No attempt should be made to reduce the angle by moving the fixation further from the eyes until the patient can undertake bar-reading at the initial fixation distance (see also Chapter 12 for further details).

Some of these cases have a convergence excess element also. This makes the above method more difficult or impossible. In some of these cases, binocular vision for near fixation can be established by an addition to the glasses for near vision as described below. Other cases need referral.

(3) *Convergence excess:* in some squints, there is a high AC/A ratio so that an abnormally high degree of convergence is associated with accommodation for near vision. This results in a squint which is either present for near vision only or in which the angle is increased markedly for near fixation. These cases should be assessed with the static distance correction in place to eliminate the accommodative element and distinguish it from the convergence excess. Where the squint is only present for near fixation and there is binocular vision for distance vision, a binocular positive addition to the correction is likely to relieve the deviation for near vision. The appropriate addition is found by trying +2 DS and applying the cover test. If there is still a deviation, the spheres can be increased. The addition which relieves the deviation is prescribed in the form of large segment bifocals with the segment top set on datum. Simultaneous vision exercises for near vision, such as bar-reading can be given to overcome suppression and establish binocular vision. Over the next several years, the addition can be reduced gradually as the binocular vision becomes more stable. In some cases, it can be discarded in time.

NON-REFRACTIVE

In many squint cases, the refractive correction does not change the angle of the deviation. In these cases, whether to prescribe glasses depends on factors other than deviation. Some have a high refractive error and require glasses to relieve symptoms of headache in hyperopia or blurred vision in myopia and astigmatism. Where there is anisometropia sufficient to blur the vision of one eye more than the other, a prescription will be needed as part of the management of any sensory adaptations. However, care must be taken in older children that the correction does not produce intractable diplopia. It is not helpful to overcome the amblyopia and suppression if single binocular vision can be restored.

Esotropia

Some convergent squint occurs following an associated event. This can be an illness such as one of the childhood illnesses which can be caught in the first few years at school. This type of squint can usually be treated by correcting any refractive error, and strengthening the prism vergences by the type of exercise described in Chapter 8. These patients have had binocular vision prior to the illness, and if they are seen soon after the recovery in general health, the binocular vision can be restored. However, care must be taken to be sure that the squint was not present before the illness as parents are not always certain on this.

In some cases, the onset of the squint may follow emotional trauma. These cases are very much more difficult to treat as the traumatic scars do not have any optometric treatment and recovery from them may be very slow. Caution should be exercised before any treatment is given. A refractive correction and prism vergence exercises may help, but the treatment may be very protracted.

Some esotropia may apparently occur spontaneously in children over the age of one year. A careful check for pathology must be carried out. This requires an ophthalmoscopic check for the white patches on the fundus indicative of retinoblastoma. This is rare but serious, and where central areas of the fundus are involved, a squint may be the first sign. It usually occurs before the age of 4 years. The ophthalmoscopy should be carried out with a dilated pupil; possibly during the cycloplegic examination (see Chapter 14). Other neurological disorders usually produce non-comitant deviations so that a motility test is essential. A sixth nerve palsy is the most likely. This will show as a restriction of abduction, and an increase in the angle of the squint as the patient looks temporally.

Non-accommodative esotropia with a spontaneous onset can occur without such pathology. It usually occurs intermittently at first. If it can be detected at this stage, developing base-in prism vergences can help to check it. A spectacle correction may not be required unless there is a significant anisometropia which may lead to amblyopia. When these squints have become established for several years, non-surgical treatment may not be successful. Prism relief may assist. The prism that gives no movement on the cover test is left in place for 10 minutes to see if the prism relief is sustained or if the deviation adapts to the prism so that the eye returns to the deviated position with the prism in place. Sometimes prism adaptation takes a week rather than 10 minutes, so that caution needs to be exercised before expecting that a prism will be a long-term solution.

Exotropia

Divergent squint can be classified under four headings, there being a different management and prognosis for each type.

(1) *Divergence excess:* presents typically as an intermittent divergent squint for distance vision only. It becomes most apparent during periods of inattention and day-dreaming, and is worse during ill health. Bright sunlight also increases the time for which the squint is present. Most patients are female, and there is little refractive error. Because of its intermittent nature, the acuities are usually good and nearly equal. There are usually no symptoms as there are sensory adaptations when the eye is deviated. Patients usually seek advice because some relative tells them that one eye goes into a corner sometimes (see also Chapter 6). Where the V syndrome exists, optometric treatment may be more difficult.

The condition is usually improved by orthoptic treatment designed to overcome the suppression and to build up the base-out prism vergences. Also useful are exercises to teach an appreciation of physiological diplopia and the movement of the diplopic images during changes of fixation from near to distance and back. This condition is also discussed in Chapter 6.

(2) *Near vision exotropia:* this is also called 'convergence insufficiency type' squint. The onset is usually in the mid-teens when binocular vision breaks down for near fixation. It seems that binocular vision has been maintained by the high convergence impulses which exist in children, but in these cases it cannot be

sustained for near when these impulses lessen. Binocular vision may also break down for distance vision but the angle of the squint is greater for near.

These patients complain of symptoms including diplopia. They are usually myopic, and have equal acuities.

If the angle is over 20^{Δ}, it is not possible to restore binocular vision by optometric methods, and the patient should be referred for a surgeon's advice. In other cases, treatment may not be lasting. The approach is to correct the refractive error, and increase the base-out prism vergences. With smaller angles, prism relief is also useful.

(3) *Basic constant exotropia:* in these cases, there is a constant divergent squint of equal angle for distance and near vision. It is often alternating with nearly equal acuities. As the onset is likely to be very early in life, there are no symptoms.

The refractive error is corrected. In children young enough to have an adequate amplitude of accommodation, the effect of prescribing negative additions to the prescription can be tried. This may eliminate the deviation, and exercises for simultaneous binocular vision may establish binocular vision. This is unlikely in children over the age of 7 years. The negative sphere incorporated in the prescription must be high enough to demonstrate no squint on the cover test. It should be gradually phased out on each successive prescription over several years. However, divergent squint is sometimes accompanied by a vertical component which will make orthoptic treatment more difficult. Patients may be better with surgical correction for cosmetic reasons.

(4) *Consecutive exotropia:* there are a number of circumstances in which a convergent squint may become divergent. It is often seen in patients who had accommodative or partially accommodative convergent squints on which an operation was performed in early childhood. No spectacles have been worn but in the mid or late teens these patients develop symptoms due to the hyperopia. Correction of the refractive error relieves the facultative accommodation and an intermittent squint with diplopia occurs. A partial correction and base-out prism vergence exercises can sometimes help to maintain binocular vision. Other cases need remedial surgery.

While the above is not a comprehensive list of all types of comitant squint, it is intended to cover those most frequently seen in optometric practice. An indication of the type of approach in dealing with these has been given in summary form. The details of orthoptic treatment for sensory adaptations is given in the preceding chapters. No line of treatment is appropriate to all squints: some need management by optometrists, some need surgery, and some will not respond whatever is done.

Reference

MOORE, S. and COHEN, R. L. (1985). Congenital exotropia: *American Orthoptic Journal,* **35,** 68–70

Part IV

Incomitant deviations

16

Investigation of comitancy

Nature of incomitant deviations

In some deviations, squint or heterophoria, the angle or degree of the deviation will vary as the patient moves the eyes to look in different parts of the field. Such deviations are incomitant. There is a consistency in the way the angle changes, so that it is increased in one particular direction of gaze for any particular patient each time the eyes are turned in that direction. It also follows that the angle of the deviation will differ according to which eye is fixing. Incomitant deviations are usually caused by abnormalities in the anatomy of the ocular motor apparatus or by particular muscles being unable to function normally. These deviations can either be present from birth, i.e. congenital, or may be acquired at any age:

(1) *Congenital* incomitancy is due to some developmental anomaly of the motor system, either in the anatomy or in the functioning of the muscles or the parts of the nervous system that serve them. This type of deviation gradually becomes more comitant as the patient gets older, but is very much less likely to respond to orthoptic treatment than comitant (or concomitant) deviations.
(2) *Acquired* incomitant deviations are caused by injury or disease of the ocular motor system. For example, they may be the result of a fracture of the skull, or of pathology affecting the muscles, nerves or brain centres. Such conditions may be long-standing, static and requiring no urgent medical attention, or can be due to recently acquired injury or active disease process. In the latter case, the patient needs referral for immediate medical attention to the ocular condition or to the disease causing the anomaly.

The complete loss of action of a muscle is called a 'muscle paralysis'. A partial loss is referred to as 'paresis' or 'muscle palsy'. In muscle palsy, the deviation usually increases in angle as the patient tries to turn the eyes into a more peripheral position of gaze, and the movement of the affected eye becomes slower. If there is a mechanical restriction of movement, the eyes may turn almost normally and quite quickly and then stop, since they are restricted from further movement.

In incomitant deviations of all kinds, non-medical treatment is very limited in remedying the patient's deviation. The first priority is to recognize those cases which require urgent medical attention. In the case of the long-standing static cases, referral should also be considered unless the patient has already been discharged after medical treatment or investigation.

A spectacle correction may be required by the patient, but it may have no effect on the deviation.

Investigation

The rest of this chapter is concerned with the detection of incomitant deviations and the interpretation of their significance. The majority of patients in need of urgent medical attention have symptoms of a kind that are likely to mean that they will take medical advice in the first place rather than consult other practitioners. It is, however, important to be able to detect incomitancy, as it will not respond at all well to orthoptics and occasionally cases of active pathology present themselves, and it is essential to be able to recognize them.

Normally, the first indication of incomitancy will emerge during a routine examination, and this may lead us to carry out additional tests to confirm the diagnosis. The sections of the routine and the additional tests are reviewed below.

History and symptoms

Incomitant deviations due to recent injury or to active pathology nearly always have a sudden and dramatic onset of symptoms – sudden diplopia being the most usual. In long-standing deviations, the symptoms are seldom so disturbing to the patient, and of course they are usually reported as having been present for as long as the deviation. The following symptoms may be present:

(1) *Diplopia* is present in most incomitancy. The patient may be able to recognize the variation in the degree of doubling in different direction of gaze. There is usually a vertical element in the diplopia. In long-standing cases, it may be intermittent due to suppression having intervened.
(2) *Abnormal head posture* may accompany the deviation; the patient may be aware of this, and may report that the abnormal head position helps in overcoming the double vision.
(3) *Blurred vision* may be present if the condition involves the third cranial nerve which also serves the ciliary muscle. For the same reason, the pupil reflexes may be abnormal.
(4) *Other symptoms* due to the disease causing the incomitant deviation may be present; for example, headache in intracranial conditions, neoplasms, vascular disturbances, etc. The diseases most likely to be associated with incomitant deviations are dealt with in a later section of this chapter, where their symptoms are also described in summary.
(5) *General health deterioration* may also occur in accompanying metabolic disorders: loss of weight, increased appetite, general fatigue, loss of muscular ability, muscular tremor, breathlessness, etc.
(6) *Injury* to the head or orbital regions may be reported, and this could cause damage to the muscular apparatus, intracranial bruising, damage or pressure from haemorrhage. This can be recent or be the explanation of a long-standing incomitant deviation. In some cases, the patient may not have thought the injury serious enough to seek medical advice at the time. Injury during the

LTL

birth delivery sometimes causes lateral rectus palsy. An operation for a previous squint can sometimes cause a degree of incomitancy.

External examination of the eyes

General inspection may show an obvious squint. Scars or asymmetry of the orbital region may indicate previous injury. Some eye-signs of systemic disease may be seen in conditions which are sometimes accompanied by squint: exophthalmos, ciliary injection, ptosis, etc.

Ophthalmoscopy

The internal examination of the eyes may also provide further evidence of pathology such as those present in vascular conditions or metabolic disease.

Motility

The examination of ocular motility is an essential part of the detection of incomitancy. Eye movements are observed as the eyes follow a fixation target such as a pentorch, which is moved in different directions of gaze in the motor field. The patient is asked to report any diplopia. The practitioner watches the eyes as they move from the primary position into each direction of the binocular field and into the extremities of the monocular periphery. This allows a subjective, and an objective, check that

(a) both eyes move smoothly and follow the target;
(b) there is a corresponding lid movement accompanying the vertical eye movements;
(c) there is no restriction of the movement of one eye in any direction of gaze.

The details of procedure for investigating the motility in routine examination are given in Chapter 2. This chapter is mainly concerned with determining the significance of any anomaly and with any additional tests which may give further information. The site of a muscle palsy can be determined from an understanding of the actions of the extrinsic ocular muscles.

The basis of muscle actions arise from one fundamental detail of their anatomy (this is shown in *Figure 16.1* which gives a scale plan view of the orbit). The eye is in the primary position, so that the visual axis is parallel to the medial wall of the orbit. The centre of rotation of the eye is marked. *Figure 16.1(a)* shows that the centre of the attachment of the superior rectus muscle is medial to the plane containing the visual axis. Although this muscle's attachment is neither symmetrical nor quite central, its general line of pull is slightly nasal to the plane containing the centre of rotation. This means that it does not act vertically over the centre of rotation. The secondary actions of this muscle can be appreciated if this fact is kept in mind: the line of pull lies medial to the centre of rotation. By reference to *Figure 16.1(a)*, it can be seen that the primary action must be to elevate the eye, and the secondary actions are adduction and intorsion. The secondary action will increase on adduction.

On abduction of the eye, the attachment of the muscle will move outwards, and the line of pull will be carried directly over the centre of rotation when the eye is abducted by about 25°. In this position, two factors are obvious: the secondary actions can no longer occur, and the primary action will be at its greatest mechanical advantage. When the eye is turned out, the superior rectus muscle will be a pure elevator and at its maximum power as an elevator; (see *Figure 16.2*).

A similar state of affairs applies to the depressor action of the inferior rectus muscle, as this lies very nearly in the same vertical plane as the superior rectus. When the eye is turned out by about 25°, the inferior rectus has its strongest action as a depressor and has no secondary actions.

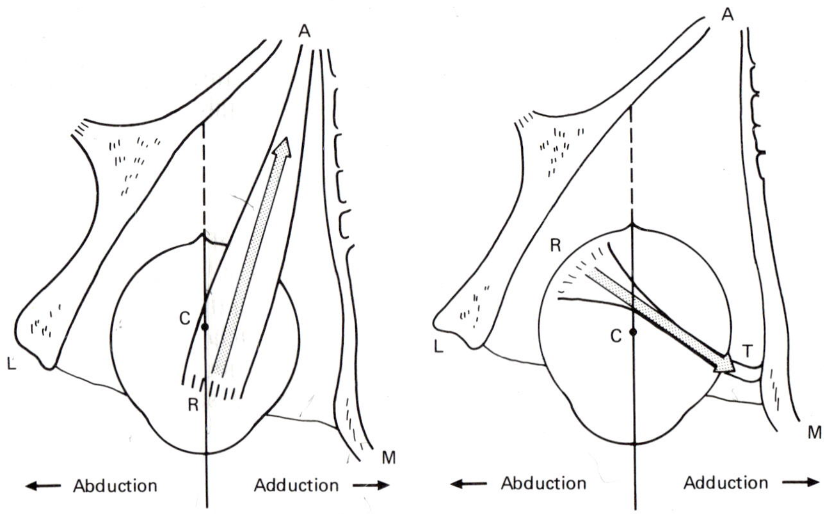

(*a*) (*b*)

Figure 16.1. Plan view of right orbit. (a) The plane and direction of pull of the superior and inferior recti muscles, RA, which passes medial to the plane of the centre of rotation of the eye. (b) The plane containing the superior and inferior oblique muscles and their direction of pull is almost the same. It passes behind and medial to the centre of rotation

The oblique muscles are shown in *Figure 16.1(b)*. From its attachment to the eye, the superior oblique pulls towards the trochlea. The line of pull is also medial to the centre of rotation, and its actions, intorsion, depression and abduction follow from this one anatomical detail. Also, as the eye turns inwards its vertical action (depression) is increased and the secondary actions are very much reduced. If the eye were to be adducted by about 55°, the line of pull would lie in the same plane as the centre of rotation. In this position, its power as a depressor would be maximum, and it would have no secondary actions.

From the point of view of clinical diagnosis, we can regard the inferior oblique muscle as lying in the same vertical plane as the superior oblique. Its actions can therefore be deduced in a similar way.

The single anatomical detail from which the muscle actions arise is that the two vertical planes containing the lines of pull of the vertical acting pairs of muscles cross medially to the centre of rotation of the eye. Once this is understood, not only can the primary and secondary actions of these muscles be deduced, but also incomitant deviation can be analysed.

Figure 16.2 shows the interaction of the two elevator muscles – the superior rectus and the inferior oblique. The central diagram shows the eye turned upwards from the primary position. Its elevation is maintained by the combined actions of both these muscles. Their individual contributions to the maintenance of elevation is shown in the vector construction above the central diagram. The diagrams on the left of the figure show the way these two muscles contribute to elevation when the eye is turned outwards (abducted), and those on the right show the contribution of each when the eye is turned inwards (adducted). In the vector construction, the sloping line SR shows how the power of the superior rectus to elevate the eye is at its maximum when the eye is abducted, and declines as the eye moves across the top of the motor field to the adducted position. The other sloping line IO indicates that the reverse is true of the oblique muscle; its elevating power is at a minimum when the eye is abducted and increases as the eye adducts. One muscle gradually

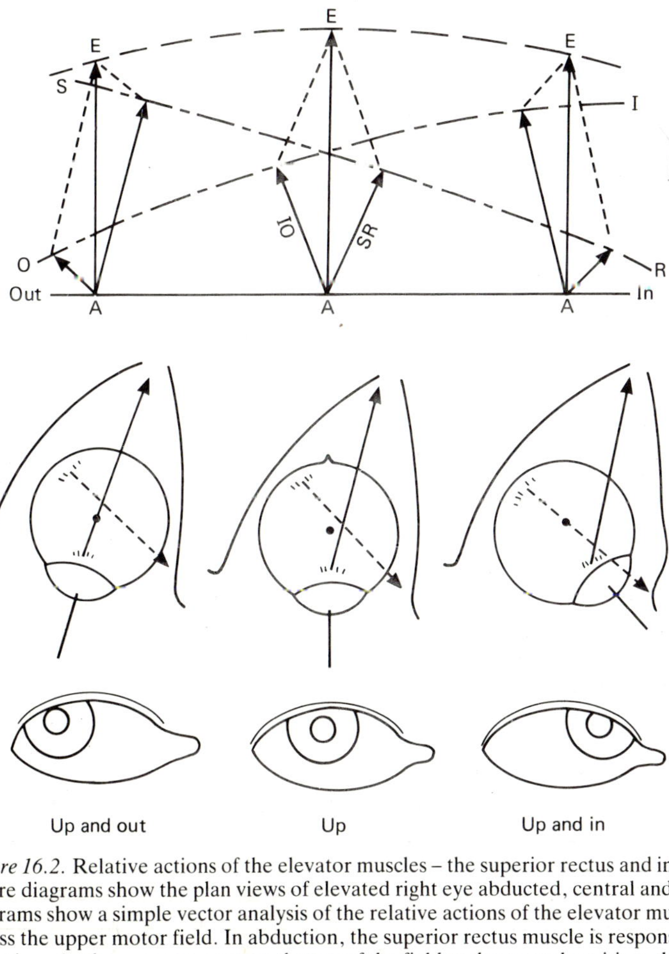

Figure 16.2. Relative actions of the elevator muscles – the superior rectus and inferior oblique. The centre diagrams show the plan views of elevated right eye abducted, central and adducted. The upper diagrams show a simple vector analysis of the relative actions of the elevator muscles as the eye moves across the upper motor field. In abduction, the superior rectus muscle is responsible for maintaining elevation. As the eye moves across the top of the field to the central position, the power of the superior rectus declines while that of the inferior oblique increases. In the adducted position, the inferior oblique maintains the elevation and the elevating power of the superior rectus is at a minimum

takes over from the other as the eye moves across the top of the field. *Figure 16.3* shows a similar treatment of the depressor muscles – the inferior rectus and the superior oblique – as the eye moves across the lower motor field in the depressed positions.

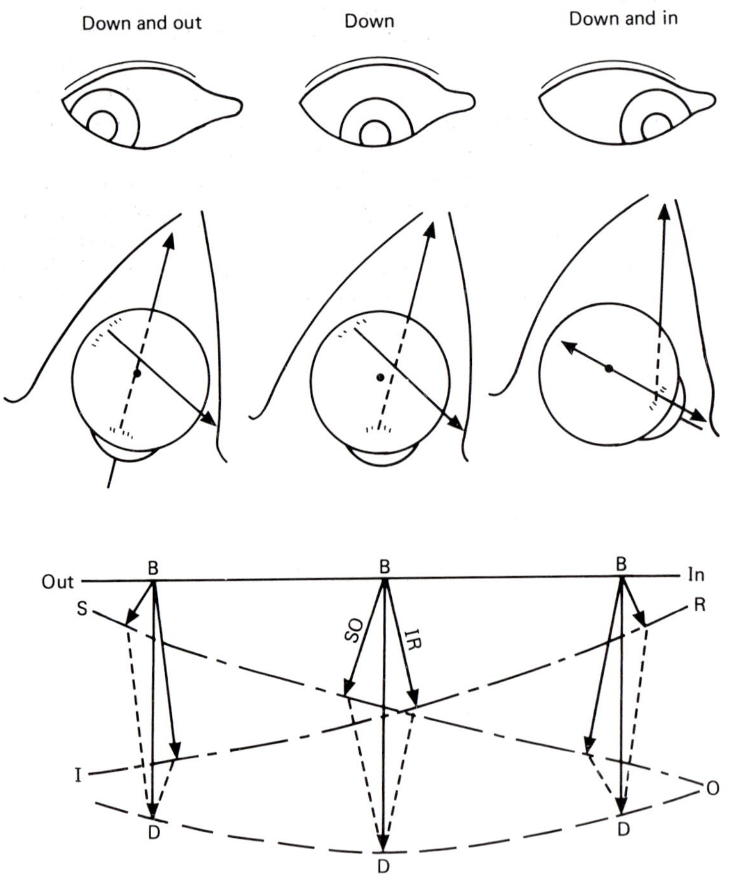

Figure 16.3. The relative actions of the depressor muscles – the inferior rectus and superior oblique: the centre diagrams show the right orbit in plan view and the lower diagrams a simple vector analysis indicating the relative strengths of the depressor muscles as the eye moves in the lower motor field

This is a slightly simplified analysis from which the clinical examination of ocular motility can be understood. A palsy or malfunction of one muscle will show as a failure of the eye to turn fully in the direction for which the muscle has the greatest mechanical advantage and therefore should have the greatest power to turn the eye. For example, a palsy of the superior oblique muscle will be detected by the restricted movement when an attempt is made to turn the eye down and inwards (see the diagram on the right-hand side of *Figure 16.3*).

It can also be noted that as the primary functions of the vertically acting muscles decrease, their secondary functions increase slightly. Thus, when the eye is turned down and inwards, the inferior rectus is pulling nearly at right-angles to the visual axis and plays little part in depression. However, its ability to adduct the eye is increased as is its ability to cyclorotate the eye (intorsion) – see *Figure 16.3*.

The medial rectus muscle in each orbit is an adductor with little secondary function, and the lateral rectus is an abductor with little other function.

In the motility test, the patient is asked to keep the head still and to follow, with the eyes, a pentorch as it is moved into the different parts of the visual motor field. Any failure of individual muscles, or group of muscles, can be assessed. The fixation light is first moved up and down in the median plane, so that the vertical eye movement and the lid movements can be observed. The light is then moved across the field at three levels: at the top, at eye level and in the lower part of the motor field. This method provides a more satisfactory result than other ways of target movement (Boylan and Clement, 1987). This is done with the patient following the light with both eyes, so that one eye's position can be judged relative to the other. A failure of one eye to follow the light in the top of the field indicates an anomaly of one of the elevators. To the patient's right and top, the affected

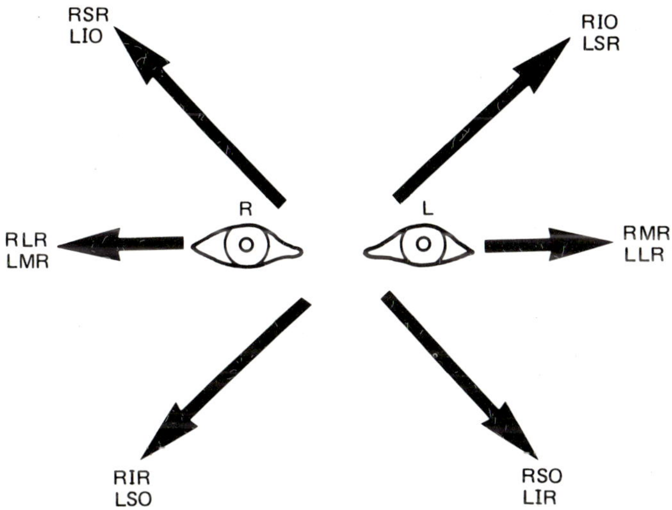

Figure 16.4. The six cardinal diagnostic positions of gaze, indicating the muscles which should have maximum power to maintain the eyes in these directions

muscle is likely to be either the right superior rectus or the left inferior oblique. Failure of one eye to turn to the right or to the left at eye level is likely to show an anomaly of either medial recti muscles or either lateral recti, and failure in the lower field shows a problem with one of the depressor muscles (see *Figure 16.4*; it should be noted that this figure does not show muscle actions, but the directions in which the elevator or depressor actions of the muscles are isolated from the other actions). In these directions of gaze, each muscle has little or no secondary actions.

The motility test is the only objective method available for standard clinical investigation of muscle paresis; photographic and electrophysiological methods require more sophisticated equipment. Small deviations of one eye when it is in a tertiary position are not easy to detect. Observation of the corneal reflection of the fixation light will help, as will the symmetry of the lid and eye positions comparing dextroversion with laevoversion. Fortunately, from the detection point of view, underaction of a muscle is usually accompanied by an overaction in the paired synergic muscle which exaggerates the angle.

Patients with active pathology nearly always have diplopia and this helps the detection. Very small degrees of diplopia may be detected subjectively, which makes diagnosis more certain. During the motility test, therefore, the patient must be asked to report any doubling and how this varies in different parts of the field. Subjective analysis of ocular motility can be assisted by the use of red and green diplopia goggles. A red goggle is worn before the right eye and a green one before the left. This assists the recognition of the images for each eye and produces slight dissociation, but the use of the goggles prevents the eyes being observed objectively.

Sometimes it is useful to be able to record the degree to which a deviation is incomitant, so that any change can be monitored to assess if the condition is getting better or worse. This can be done by several methods.

THE MADDOX GROOVE OR HAND FRAME

This can be used to measure the deviation in different directions of gaze. Using the Maddox groove and a pentorch, the patient's head is kept still while measurements are taken in different parts of the field. It is important that the light is at a fixed distance and is moved to definite peripheral positions, so that the test is repeatable. It is suggested that it is held at 50 cm from the eyes, and at the corners of a square formation in front of the patient and of 50 cm dimension.

THE COVER TEST

This can be similarly applied, and the eye movement neutralized by prisms in the fixed peripheral positions as well as with the eyes in the primary position.

HESS SCREEN METHODS

These methods provide another way of recording the degree of incomitancy and other information which will help the assessment of the progress of the condition. Modern screens are grey in colour, so that the light from two projector torches can be seen on the screen. The patient sits at a distance of 50 cm. The screen is marked in 'squares' representing 5° rotations of the eyes. As the screen is flat, tangential to the line of sight, the squares are distorted into a pincushion pattern. The practitioner holds the red torch and the patient wears red/green diplopia goggles. On the screen, the red image from this torch can be seen only by the eye with the red goggle before it. Thus, when the patient is asked to look at the red bar image on the screen, the eye will be positioned so that the red image falls on the fovea of that eye. The patient holds the green torch and is asked to shine its bar image on the screen so that it appears to cross the red bar. This subjective cross will be formed when the green bar of light is in such a position that its image falls on the fovea, as the fovea in each eye are corresponding points and have the same visual direction. Therefore, the positions of the bar images on the screen mark the points on intersection of the visual axes with the screen. The degree of any deviation can be estimated from the 5° marking. If the deviation varies as the red fixation bar is moved from one position to another, an incomitant deviation is demonstrated. If the goggles are changed round so that the red goggle is in front of the other eye, the plot can be repeated with this eye fixing and the first one deviated. A copy of the chart is made on a paper chart with each eye fixing in turn (see *Figure 16.5*).

The Foster, the Lancaster and the Lees screens all share the same general principle as the Hess screen, but have a different mechanical set-up.

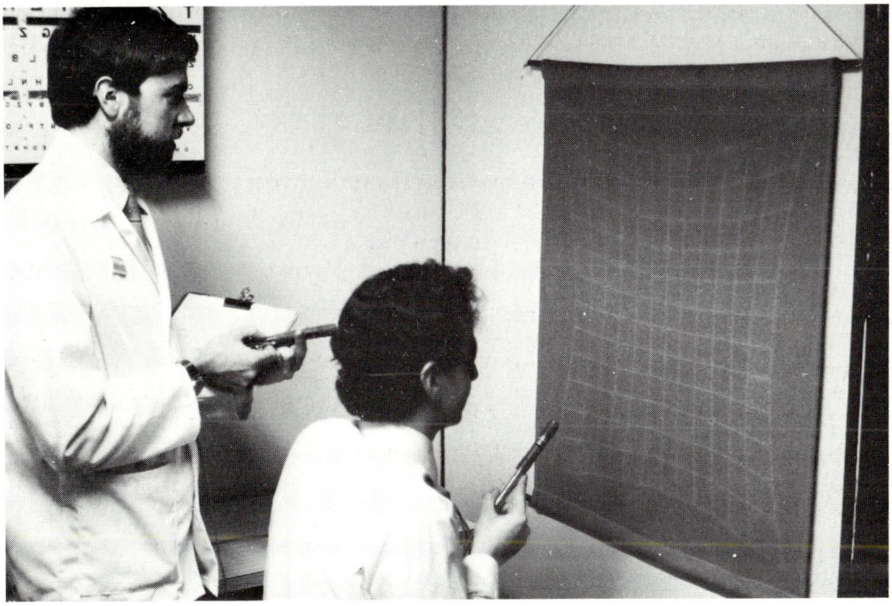

Figure 16.5. The Hess screen in use – a simple felt screen with Foster torches

The interpretation of the Hess screen plot is assisted by remembering that the smaller of the two plots will be that from the affected eye, and that the greatest underaction will normally be in the field of the primary affected muscle. A Hess screen analysis may also appear to indicate the following sequence:

(a) the primary muscle palsy shows as the greatest underaction;
(b) overaction of the contralateral synergic muscle – this will increase the apparent size of the deviation;
(c) a contracture, failure to relax, of the direct antagonist which will show as an overaction;
(d) a secondary inhibitional palsy of the contralateral antagonist which shows as an underaction in the field of this muscle.

Eyelid signs

Abnormalities of the lids may sometimes be useful in indicating the presence of an incomitant deviation. The width of the palpebral fissure should be noted:

(1) In the primary position of the eyes when the right and left lid openings are compared. The width may be judged by the amount of the limbus visible through the lid openings. An abnormally wide fissure (Dalrymple's sign of thyrotoxicosis) may be accompanied by hypophoria or hypotropia which

increases on elevation of the eyes. Ptosis and diplopia, which are both worse at the end of the day, can be an early sign of myasthenia gravis – a rare muscle disease. Ptosis can also be a sign of third nerve palsy. A hypotropic position of one eye may show a 'pseudo-ptosis'; the lid is slightly lower as the eye is turned down.

(2) During the motility test, a lag of the lids on downward gaze (von Graefe's sign) may be present in thyrotoxicosis. A change in lid fissure, when looking left or right, occurs in Duane's retraction syndrome, which is an anomaly of the lateral rectus (see later).

Abnormal head postures

An habitual abnormal head posture may be a sign of a number of things, such as congenital shortening of a neck muscle (torticollis), nystagmus, a field restriction, unilateral deafness, shyness, or just habit. It can be a sign of an incomitant deviation, in which case it can be thought of as having one or more of three components:

(1) *Facial turn* – if the face is turned either to the left or to the right, this can be a sign of an anomaly of a medial or lateral rectus muscle. For example, diplopia may be avoided in right lateral rectus palsy by turning the face to the right so that contraction of the right lateral rectus is not required.
(2) *Chin raised or lowered* – this may occur in A or V syndromes. The deviation in these cases may be quite small or absent in upwards gaze, so that the patient habitually carries the head with the chin down to avoid diplopia: A pattern. In the V syndrome, the reverse may be true, so that the head position may be an important diagnostic clue in these cases. For further details of A and V syndromes, see later.
(3) *Head tilt* – if binocular vision is present in part or all of the motor field, the head may be tilted to make it easier to avoid diplopia or to extend the area of single vision. The head tilt may be combined with a facial turn and raised or lowered chin. The direction of the tilt may be determined in the interests of levelling the diplopic images to assist fusion, or to compensate for the loss of cyclorotation of one eye if there is paresis of one of the oblique muscles. The most frequently seen head tilt occurs in superior oblique palsy. The face is turned away from the affected eye, the chin turned down and the head tilted away from the affected side.

In long-standing deviations, the abnormal head position becomes less obvious. The absence of an abnormal position of the head does not mean that the deviation is comitant.

Localization disturbances

The localization of objects in space is determined visually by a combination of two mechanisms: retinal localization, and the motor system's directional mechanism. The position of the image on the retina determines the direction in which it is perceived – its visual location. Because the eyes and head move, the brain must also take these movements into account in localizing an object with respect to the egocentre. Eccentric fixation can cause a disturbance of the retinal system when the fixation point moves away from the centre of localization at the fovea: past pointing occurs (see Chapter 11). Also, if the eyes do not move correctly in response to the nerve impulses sent to the muscles, as in paretic squint, the motor localization system will be disturbed.

The past pointing test may also be used to demonstrate these motor disturbances. The test is applied monocularly to each eye in turn, as described in Chapter 11. Past pointing will be demonstrated in the eye having the affected muscle and the field of action of this muscle. The degree of past pointing will increase as the eye turns further into the direction of its action, and will not occur in the opposite direction of gaze. This test can be made more effective by holding a card horizontally at the level of the patient's chin, so that it occludes the patient's pointing hand from view while the target appears above the card. Past pointing only occurs with paresis of recent onset, and lessens as the patient adapts to the deviation.

Evaluation

The first priority with incomitant deviations is to decide if there is an active pathological cause requiring immediate medical attention, or if it is a long-standing deviation. *Table 16.1* summarizes the factors that help in this evaluation.

TABLE 16.1. Summary of main factors to be considered in assessing incomitant deviations for active pathology

Factor	*Congenital or long-standing*	*Recent onset*
Diplopia	Unusual	Always present in at least one direction of gaze
Onset	Patient does not know when the deviation began	Sudden and distressing
Ambylopia	Often present	Absent
Comitance	More comitant with time	Always incomitant
Abnormal head posture	Slight, but persists on covering paretic eye	More marked; the patient is aware of it: disappears on covering paretic eye
Past pointing	Absent	Present
Other symptoms	Unlikely	May be present due to the primary cause

It will be seen that one of the differences between deviations of recent pathological cause and more long-standing deviations is that there may be other symptoms of the general pathological condition. It is therefore useful to be aware of the primary conditions which can give rise to incomitant deviations and of the other signs and symptoms that may accompany them. There is a very large number of these conditions. They include infections of the nervous system, metabolic disorders, vascular lesions, neoplasms, toxins and trauma to the head and orbital regions. Some of these may have incomitant diplopia as an early sign before the patient is really aware of the seriousness of other signs and symptoms. This is not a very frequent occurrence, but that means we must be all the more vigilant and continue to bear in mind the possibility. In other conditions, the deviation may occur as part of the possible progress of the disease for which the patient is already under treatment. The patient's medical adviser needs to be made aware of this development.

Some of the most common of the conditions which may have ocular muscle palsy as an early sign or as part of the progress of the condition are described below. The other general symptoms that can accompany the diplopia are also given as a means of helping to confirm the diagnosis of the deviation as of recent pathological cause.

(1) *Diabetes* – ocular palsy is found in about one-third of diabetic patients. It usually affects the third cranial nerve (third nerve palsy), and may sometimes affect the pupil reflex and reduce the amplitude of the accommodation. There are two groups of patients: young patients between 15 and 20 years of age with severe diabetes of sudden onset, and older sufferers of 55 years and over who have a more gradual onset. The symptoms of diabetes may include, in addition to the diplopia, generalized headache in most of the older age group, increased thirst and urination, increased appetite with loss of weight, constipation, boils or other skin conditions. The older patients are mostly overweight females.

(2) *Thyrotoxicosis* – this can occur with muscle palsy. There is usually difficulty in elevation of the eyes which can appear to be a superior rectus palsy, but in fact more than one muscle may be affected regardless of the nerve paths. This is because the muscle tissue itself may be affected; most frequently the inferior rectus is changed in such a way that it will not stretch to allow the eye to elevate (a contracture). Exophthalmos may be present, but not invariably. Other signs can include von Graefe's sign, retraction of the upper lid, infrequent blinking, conjunctival injection (red eye), vertical diplopia, and sometimes poor near point of convergence. This condition occurs most often in females over 40 years of age, and may be accompanied by increased appetite and loss of weight, clammy hands and tremor of the outstretched hand.

(3) *Hypertension* – the chances of hypertension being accompanied by ocular palsy increases with age as the blood supply to the cranial nerves becomes involved. In addition to the vascular changes seen on the fundus, symptoms may include headache, dizziness, breathlessness and ringing in the ears.

(4) *Aneurysms* – the ocular palsy is accompanied by frontal pain on the same side. The symptoms of hypertension may also be present.

(5) *Temporal arteritis* – marked temporal pain is present with intermittent diplopia, loss of appetite and general lassitude. The ocular palsy occurs in a minority of patients and before the loss of vision begins.

(6) *Disseminated sclerosis* – ocular palsy is an early sign in about half the patients, who are usually under 40 years. Other symptoms include the loss of muscle co-ordination, a weakness in one limb, or slurring of speech. This condition can begin with optic neuritis.

(7) *Myasthenia gravis* – this is a comparatively rare condition occurring first between the ages of 20 and 40 years. Double vision and ocular palsy is an early sign in about half the cases. This is temporary and may go away during the day. Other muscles in the body may be affected. The ocular muscle most often involved is the levator, so that ptosis is the most usual ocular sign. If the patient is asked to look downwards for 15 seconds and then quickly back to the primary position, an upward twitch of the upper lid is seen before it resumes the ptosis position (Cogan's sign).

While it is useful, in diagnosis of a pathological cause, to note some of the symptoms mentioned here, it must be remembered that many other conditions may cause incomitant deviations.

Muscle palsies

Another aspect which can help in the diagnosis of incomitant deviation is the recognition of particular muscle palsies which are given below.

FOURTH NERVE OR SUPERIOR OBLIQUE PALSY

This is fairly common as a congenital anomaly, and it may be characterized by a head tilt away from the affected side. If the patient is asked to tilt the head to the other side, the affected eye elevates (the head tilting test). The head tilt usually disappears in early adolescence, and there may be binocular vision in the primary position of the eyes.

An acquired fourth nerve palsy may occur in damage to the trochlea, as in an uppercut blow in boxing or in a blow on the crown of the head. Diplopia will be greatest when looking down and inwards, or when reading.

SIXTH NERVE OR LATERAL RECTUS PALSY

This is a common incomitant anomaly which can be the result of instrumentation during birth delivery. The long intracranial path of the sixth nerve makes it particularly susceptible to lesions acquired later. Because of the close association of the sixth and seventh cranial nerves in the mid-brain, the facial muscles also may be involved.

Lateral rectus palsy as a congenital condition produces an alternating convergent squint with equal acuities if the anomaly is bilateral. If it is unilateral, the face is turned towards the affected side.

GRADENIGO'S SYNDROME

This is a lateral rectus palsy caused by an inner ear infection, possibly during birth delivery. A unilateral incomitant convergent squint (usually the left eye) is accompanied by trigeminal pain of the face, deafness and a facial turn to the affected side. This condition has become rare since antiobiotics came into general use.

DUANE'S RETRACTION SYNDROME

In this condition, which is more frequently found in females, the affected eye behaves as if the lateral rectus muscle has been replaced by non elastic non-contractile tissue. The most usual pattern of signs (Type A) is restriction of abduction of the affected eye, whereas on adduction there is also a restriction of movement and a marked retraction of the eye back into orbit. The retraction causes pseudo-ptosis, and there may be elevation of the eye. Sometimes (Type B), the adduction is not restricted, and in other cases (Type C), the adduction is affected more than the abduction.

STRABISMUS FIXUS

This is an uncommon condition in which the medial rectus seems to be replaced by non-elastic tissue, and there is no abduction of the affected eye.

SUPERIOR OBLIQUE TENDON SHEATH (BROWN'S SYNDROME)

In this usually congenital condition, the sheath of the superior oblique muscle's tendon between the trochlea and the insertion into the globe is too short. This prevents elevation when the eye is turned inwards, giving the appearance of paresis of the inferior oblique.

BLOWOUT FRACTURE

This is an acquired anomaly due to a fracture of the floor of the orbit. As the fracture heals, orbital fascial tissue is trapped in the maxillary sinus preventing the eye from elevating above the horizontal. It is caused by a blow on the front of the face; for example, from a cricket ball or from falling on the face. There may be retraction of the eye as it tries to turn up; this can be seen from the side.

SUPERIOR RECTUS PALSY

This sometimes occurs as a congenital isolated muscle palsy and is usually accompanied by ptosis.

The medial and inferior recti and inferior oblique muscles are seldom affected as congenital isolated anomalies, but may be involved with other muscles.

THIRD NERVE PALSY OR OPHTHALMOPLEGIA

If all the extrinsic muscles supplied by the third cranial are affected together, the condition is known as 'complete oculomotor palsy'. If only the extrinsic muscles supplied by this nerve are affected, this is external ophthalmoplegia. A paresis of the ciliary muscle and the iris sphincter is known as internal ophthalmoplegia, and when both the extrinsic and intrinsic muscles are affected, there is total ophthalmoplegia. In the last condition, there will be a divergent squint with slightly depressed eyes, ptosis and a loss of pupil action and accommodation. Other accompanying symptoms may include headache, a tremor of the contralateral limbs (due to the involvement of the red nucleus where the third nerve fibres pass), and other symptoms of diabetes (see above). Ophthalmoplegia can also be due to a blow on the frontal region of the head.

GAZE PALSIES

These can occur due to lesions in the frontal motor centre, gaze centres in the pons or in the interconnecting pathways. There is seldom diplopia, and the eyes move together in most directions of gaze. In one direction, the eyes cannot move reflexly to take up fixation or, more rarely, cannot follow a moving target (pursuit palsy). In lateral gaze palsy, the two eyes will not move beyond the mid-line. In vertical gaze palsy, movements above the horizontal are restricted, or there is no vertical movement at all; rarely there is no downward movement.

A AND V SYNDROMES

These may be regarded as incomitant deviations. In the A syndrome, the eyes are more convergent on upward gaze and more divergent on depression. Therefore, in eso-deviations there may be binocular fixation in downwards gaze and a squint when the patient looks upwards. The opposite is true for exo-deviations. In the V pattern, the eyes are more divergent on elevation and less on depression. These patterns may be present as congenital anomalies, or may accompany an acquired squint, particularly where the oblique muscles are affected.

Management

Considerable attention has been given in this chapter to the diagnosis of conditions requiring medical attention. This is obviously the first priority in the interest of the patient. The number of patients who have incomitant deviations as an early sign of disease requiring urgent medical attention is not large, and many of them will take medical advice in the first place. This means that the largest number of incomitant deviations likely to be seen will be long-standing deviations, and most of these will already have had medical attention. Therefore, the question which arises is whether there is anything further that can be done in these long-standing cases. Incomitant deviations do not respond at all well to orthoptic procedures. Very occasionally, congenital conditions in children may be helped by exercises to extend the area of the binocular field over which there is binocular vision, or to re-establish it when it has broken down due to general ill-health. In the latter case, the patient may suddenly experience double vision, which may be remedied by orthoptic exercises if it is established that the general condition has cleared.

Patients with long-standing deviations will have suppression which prevents diplopia over most of the visual field. There may be some diplopia in one peripheral part of the motor field. Usually it is better not to disturb this adapted or partially adapted state. If one eye has been neglected or has had a blurred image for many years, correcting the refractive error can well produce troublesome diplopia. It may be better to give a balancing lens or a blurring lens to maintain the status quo. In some cases, correction may be appropriate, particularly in children, if it is likely that some binocular vision can be restored perhaps with relieving prisms. However, this is a difficult procedure, and should only be attempted with great caution. Once diplopia is created, it is difficult for the patient to revert to suppression. Very occasionally, the sensory adaptation in these incomitant deviations seems to break down spontaneously, and we are presented with a patient complaining of diplopia and a long-standing deviation not due to recently acquired pathology. Prisms may be prescribed to extend the area of single vision. These need to be a compromise, as the deviation increases as the eye turns more peripherally, but the aim is to give prism relief for the central part of the motor field. Try prism of the power of the deviation shown by a Maddox groove with the eyes in the primary position. Carry out the cover test to see if this gives recovery when the occluder is removed, first with the eyes in the primary position, and then with the fixation increasing further into the part of the motor field most affected. A judgement needs to be made in each case as to how strong a prism is reasonable in terms of weight and edge thickness, and how much peripheral vision can be restored. These are difficult cases. In large angles, a surgeon's opinion can be sought and prisms considered only for the residual angle after operation.

Reference

BOYLAN, C. and CLEMENT, R. A.(1987). Excursion tests of ocular motility. *Ophthalmic and Physiological Optics,* **7**(1), 31–35

Bibliography

BURIAN, H. M. and VON NOORDEN, G. K. (1974). *Binocular Vision and Ocular Motility.* Mosby, St. Louis

DALE, R. T. (1982). *Fundamentals of Ocular Motility and Strabismus.* Grune & Stratton, New York

DUKE-ELDER, SIR STEWART (1973). *System of Ophthalmology*, vol. VI, *Ocular Motility and Strabismus.* Kimpton, London

SCHEIE, M. D. and ALBERT, D. M. (1969). *Adler's Textbook of Ophthalmology*, Saunders, Philadelphia

17

Nystagmus

Smc

Nystagmus is a continued oscillation, usually of both eyes, in the form of a regular to and fro movement. It is nearly always involuntary. It can be physiological, congenital and long-standing, or a sign of the onset of neurological disease. Physiological nystagmus obviously requires no action; some help may be given in the congenital and long-standing types, but where it is the result of active disease it needs immediate referral for medical investigation.

Symptoms

The symptoms are a very important part of the investigation of nystagmus and a key factor in deciding if there is an active pathological cause. Long-standing congenital nystagmus is usually comparatively free from troublesome symptoms, whereas the recently acquired types will give rise to very disturbing subjective effects. The likely symptoms are:

(1) *Reduced acuity* – this occurs because the eyes cannot maintain fixation. There is always reduced acuity in nystagmus.
(2) *Oscillopia* – an apparent movement of the visual environment to and fro as the eyes oscillate is present in recently acquired nystagmus, but not in the long-standing types. Where it is present, it is very disturbing and is usually accompanied by dizziness.
(3) *Abnormal head posture* – as the nystagmoid movements may be less in some part of the motor field, the patient may turn the head into an abnormal position so that the eyes are turned relative to the orbits.
(4) *Past pointing* – this may be demonstrated in recently acquired nystagmus.
(5) *Diplopia* – this is experienced in many cases.

Classification of oscillation

The oscillations of the eyes should be observed to determine the type, degree, direction, amplitude and frequency; this will sometimes help in the diagnosis:

(1) *Type* – the nystagmus can be either pendular, when the speed of movement is equal in both directions, or it can be jerky if it is a slow drift in one direction followed by a fast movement back.

(2) *Degree* – the classification according to what part of the motor field is affected determines the degree.
   (a) First degree, the nystagmus is present in peripheral gaze only.
   (b) Second degree, the nystagmus is present in the primary position, but not in some other direction of gaze; an abnormal head posture is very likely.
   (c) Third degree, the nystagmus is present over all the motor field.

(3) *Direction of movement* – this can be horizontal, vertical, diagonal or rotary.

(4) *Amplitude*: (a) fine, less than 5° (the cornea moves less than 1 mm); (b) medium, 5°–10° (cornea moves about 2 or 3 mm); (c) coarse, over 10°.

(5) *Frequency* – the classification of frequency varies with different authorities, but an oscillation of 1 per sec may be regarded as slow, and over 10 per sec as fast.

Physiological types of nystagmus

Physiological types of nystagmus include the very small oscillations occurring in normal fixation and which are not visible on normal inspection; nystagmus in the very extreme of the motor field when trying to fix an object barely in the motor field of one eye; and the vertical nystagmus when the eyes are closed, which is associated with Bell's phenomenon. Nystagmus can be produced physiologically by looking at a continuous moving display, opticokinetic nystagmus, or produced by thermal or rotary stimulation of the inner ear.

Congenital types of nystagmus are usually classified in the following types.

Sensory or ocular nystagmus

This is due to something preventing the establishment of the fixation reflex in very early life; for example, albinism, some congenital cataracts and macular lesions, and optic atrophy. The nystagmus is always bilateral. In these cases, the movement is usually pendular, and the primary cause may be obvious.

Hereditary nystagmus

This seems to have an incidence of about 1 in 6500. It shows sex-linked inheritance and therefore is most frequent in males. There are usually other male members of the family with a similar condition. There is no invariable pattern but it may have the following features. The frequency and amplitude usually increase on right or on left gaze. It is jerky with the fast phase towards the direction of gaze: the eyes drift slowly away from the primary position and then jerk back as if trying to maintain fixation in the periphery. There is usually a 'null' position where the nystagmus is minimal which may be central or slightly peripheral. There may be an abnormal head posture to maintain the eyes in the null position and this is particularly noticeable when trying to read the letter chart. Occlusion of one eye accentuates the nystagmus. In about half the cases, there is also infantile esotropic syndrome (see Chapter 14). The amplitude of the nystagmus may be reduced in convergence for near vision, and it is increased when the patient is under emotional stress.

This type of nystagmus may be very serious when the patient is under 5 years of age, but as he gets older the nystagmus lessens and may completely disappear in the years following adolescence.

MANAGEMENT

These patients have usually had medical investigation previously. A correction for any refractive error may assist. Use a trial frame that allows the refraction to take place in the abnormal head position where the acuity is best: a bracket-held refractor unit is not suitable. Occlude the eye not under test by a +10 D sphere instead of an opaque occluder which may increase the nystagmus.

Prisms may help in two ways. If the oscillation is less on convergence, base-out prism may help. Similarly, prism with the base direction the same way before both eyes can sometimes relieve the abnormal head posture, but the weight and prism distortion set a limit to this.

In cases of amblyopia and squint, it may be appropriate to treat these conditions. Occlusion should not be used, but penalization methods may be appropriate.

The patient or parent may be assured that no serious sequel is likely to follow, and that the condition tends to get better rather than worse.

Latent nystagmus

In many ways this gives the appearance of a mild form of hereditary nystagmus, but the oscillations only occur when one eye is covered. The movement may be in the occluded or the unoccluded eye, or both. There is a squint in most cases, and dissociated vertical deviation may be present. Both the nystagmus and the dissociated vertical deviation may be greater if the dominant eye is covered. There is usually jerky nystagmus, with the fast movement in the direction of the covered eye.

This anomaly appears to be caused by a disturbance in the binocular visual location system: the binoculus or visual egocentre is not transferred to the unoccluded eye when the retinal illumination in one eye is decreased sufficiently to suspend vision. The condition often disappears at about the age of 20 years.

Unless it is accompanied by a squint, latent nystagmus does not cause the patient any trouble and requires no treatment. Squinting patients may be treated if other factors are favourable. Although most authorities say that occlusion for treatment of amblyopia is contraindicated, von Noorden *et al.* (1987) have found occlusion of non-amblyopic eye effective in strabismic amblyopia. During subjective refraction, a + 10D sphere should be used instead of an occluder.

Spasmus nutans

This is a transient form of nystagmus which occurs during early infancy. It is of small amplitude, pendular and fast. It usually occurs during the first year of life and recovers spontaneously in a few months. It may be accompanied by a tremulous nodding of the head. Parents sometimes ask for assurance about it.

Voluntary nystagmus

Some persons can produce a short burst of voluntary fast nystagmus. This seems to be of no clinical significance.

Pathological types of nystagmus

Neurogenic nystagmus

Lesions of any part of the motor nervous system serving eye movements may cause nystagmus: brain-stem, longitudinal bundle, or oculomotor and vestibular nuclei. It may be a sign of disseminated sclerosis, cerebral tumours, thrombosis of the inferior cerebral artery, or poisons such as carbon monoxide, chloroform, barbiturates or alcohol; sometimes it accompanies other diseases of the nervous system such as syphilis or poliomyelitis. Ophthalmoplegia may be present.

There are always disturbing symptoms, including oscillopia, reduced acuity and headache. The nystagmus is nearly always jerky, and increases in one direction of gaze. It may begin as first-degree nystagmus. Sometimes it is horizontal during horizontal eye movements and vertical during vertical movements. Its exact nature will depend on the site and cause of the lesion. It needs immediate medical investigation.

Acquired nystagmus can occur in an infant too young to report symptoms. There is usually a vertical element in the movement which may be accentuated on elevation or depression of the eyes. Where this vertical movement is noted, referral for medical investigation is indicated.

Ocular dysmetria

This is due to a lesion of the cerebellum which prevents co-ordination of muscle movements and proper orientation during movements. When it affects the eyes, dysmetria results in disturbances of conjugate movements: the eyes overshoot and have to make nystagmoid corrective movements. 'Ocular flutter' may be present; there is a rapid burst of horizontal nystagmus noticed by the patient as blurred vision. These problems are rare, but require referral.

Miners' nystagmus

This is caused by inadequate stimulation for fixation due to poor illumination over a period of 20 years or more of underground work. There may be other factors contributing to its cause. It is still seen in mining areas. The symptoms consist of oscillopia, leading to headaches and dizziness. The nystagmus is second degree, pendular or jerky, horizontal or vertical. It is usually of small amplitude and fast frequency. It increases on upward gaze, which causes the chin to be raised. If it has not already been investigated, it needs referral for possible financial compensation.

The reader is referred to books on neurology or ophthalmology for a full treatment of nystagmus. What has been given here is a general summary to enable these conditions to be recognized.

Reference

VON NOORDEN, G. K., AVILLA, C., SIDIKARO, Y. and LAROCH, R.(1987). Latent nystagmus and strabismic amblyopia. *American Journal of Ophthalmology,* **103,** 87–89

Index